JOURNEY TO THE CRIB:
A CONTEMPORARY APPROACH
TO INFERTILITY

JOURNEY TO THE CRIB: A CONTEMPORARY APPROACH TO INFERTILITY

DAVID KREINER, MD

Sunshine Publishers
1074 Old Country Road
Plainview, NY 11803

Printed in the United States of America

ISBN: 978-0-9826584-0-6

CONTENTS

Foreword.. 9

Preface.. 11

Through My Eyes: An Historical Perspective On IVF 13

THE JOURNEY BEGINS

The Pregnancy Test Is Negative Again, What Do I Do?................... 18

What Are My Odds? 21

Where Do You Go? 25

Meet The Doctor 28

CAUSES OF INFERTILIY

Have You Had A Fertility Workup?... 32

Are Fibroids and Polyps Preventing You from Getting Pregnant?...... 36

Hydrosalpinx... 39

Polycystic Ovarian Disease 41

Endometriosis 44

Endometriosis And Your Infertility.. 47

What Do You Know About Your Fertility? 51

Sperm Meets Egg – Why Doesn't It Work Every Time? 57

TREATMENT OF INFERTILITY

Trying To Conceive With Clomid Therapy 66

Intrauterine Insemination (IUI) 69

MicroIVF 71

In Vitro Fertilization and Embryo Culture 73

Medications For IVF Treatment 76

Fertility Drugs Do Not Increase Risk for Ovarian Cancer 81

Co-Culture of Embryos Offered at East Coast Fertility 86

Things You Should Know About Your Embryo Transfer................... 89

Cryopreservation of Embryos 91

WAYS TO DEAL WITH STRESS
AND OPTIMIZE PREGNANCY SUCCESS

Nominated For Best Supporting Role is… 96
I Look Pretty Good In Scrubs 98
Is This Stress Making Me Look Fat? 100
Tips for Reducing Infertility Stress 102
Fertility and the MIND & BODY connection 106
Alternative Therapies and Holistic Medicine 109

CONTEMPORARY ISSUES IN INFERTILITY

A Dozen Embryos, Who Will Stop This Madness? 112
No More "Jon and Kate" Casualties 115
Why "The Wyden Bill" Does Not Support Infertility Patients 117
Gift of Life and Its Price 121
When Are You Too Old To Be A Mother? 123
Octomom 126
Fertility doctor denounced for claims of human cloning 127
Fertility Treatment During This Economic Downturn 129

ABC's of IVF 132

DVD CONTENTS

1. Introduction to Dr. Kreiner
2. Advances in The Field
3. Single Embryo Transfer
4. MicroIVF – Part 1
5. MicroIVF – Part 2
6. High FSH and the Biological Clock
7. Financing Treatment
8. Polycystic Ovarian Syndrome
9. Fibroids
10. Egg Donation
11. Accessibility to Your Doctor
12. Polyps

JOURNEY TO THE CRIB:
A CONTEMPORARY APPROACH

THIS BOOK was written to assist patients with their personal fertility journeys. It takes the patient through the process of learning what is causing the infertility and how to find the best treatments for it. All aspects of infertility and treatments are discussed as well as contemporary newsworthy issues that have been of particular recent interest.

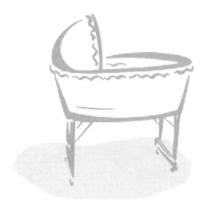

FOREWORD

JOURNEY To The Crib, A Contemporary Approach To Infertility was written for the benefit of my patients and others seeking assistance in building their families. It is my sincere hope that the information offered in this book will make your personal journey easier and more successful. Many of the chapters have accompanying videos which may make them more enjoyable and understandable. You may find that the sections on Causes and Treatment of Infertility are especially relevant if you are told that you have that particular diagnosis or if the specific treatment discussed in that chapter is recommended to you. You may find it more convenient to use the book more as a reference for subjects that pertain directly to your case.

The Contemporary Issues section includes topics on infertility and IVF that have been appearing in the newspapers and magazines during the past year. These include such issues as the risk of multiple pregnancies with infertility treatments and options to minimize risk and cost.

A glossary is added at the end for general reference and it is recommended that the reader use it as such since some of the material gets technical in nature where I occasionally use a medical language that may still be foreign to you. I apologize in advance but at least I give you a dictionary in the form of a glossary to help you follow along.

I wish you all the best of luck with your journey!

Thanks to my parents, Beatrice and Irving Kreiner who literally started me on my own journey to the crib and beyond. They have always served as an inspiration to me in my career to assist others in achieving that which they had perfected, the warm, nurturing family. Thanks to my wife, Robin and my children, Dan, Jay, Ashley and Aly as well as my daughter in law, Katy and my grandchildren; Jayden, Devon and Kaylen and to Robyn. They reinforce how wonderfully purposeful a family can make your life. It is my personal high regard for having one's own family that drives me to help others achieve the same.

PREFACE

HISTORY OF IVF

ALTHOUGH most of us think of IVF as one of the great technological advances conceived towards the end of the 20th century, records show that man has been working towards the goal of assisted conception since the 3rd century AD. Jewish thinkers discussed the possibility of accidental or unintentional human insemination by artificial means. Let us also not forget the surrogate birth of a son for Abraham who with wife Sarah had longstanding infertility issues.

In the 14th century AD there are accounts of Arabs using artificial insemination on horses. The first human artificial insemination occurred in 1785. In 1969, human fertilization was achieved and eventually embryos were developed at Columbia University which were discarded due to an ethics controversy over the process at the university.

In 1978, the first IVF birth in the world occurred in the UK with the first "test tube" baby, Louise Brown. In 1979, the American Reproductive pioneering couple Howard and Georgeanna Jones achieved the first successful IVF in the western hemisphere after a forced retirement from Johns Hopkins. They were recruited at age 65 by their old friend, Mason Andrews, who at the time was not only mayor of Norfolk, Virginia but also was chairman of obstetrics and gynecology at the new Eastern Virginia Medical School. Both Howard and Georgeanna prior to coming to Norfolk had distinguished careers in Reproductive Medicine and infertility. Over the next 10 years they established the premier IVF program in the world, teaching physicians from Asia, Europe, and South America and treating patients from all over.

I arrived in Norfolk in 1985 to initiate my fellowship training in IVF at a time when the pregnancy rate from IVF was 15%. Today, at East Coast Fertility in Long Island, our average patient has better than a 60% chance of conceiving from a single IVF stimulation and retrieval. Then we used to have to operate through a laparoscope inserted through the abdomen to retrieve the eggs. Now we do so in a 15 minute procedure by needle aspiration through the vagina. We can achieve pregnancies in menopausal women through donor egg as well as select healthy embryos in women with hereditary genetic disorders. I like to think that when I assist a couple in starting their family I am continuing the tradition and biblical commandment to be fruitful and multiply; a need intrinsic to the human condition

THROUGH MY EYES: AN HISTORICAL PERSPECTIVE ON IVF

My first day of fellowship training in Reproductive Endocrinology at the Jones Institute was the day the Institute moved from the old quarters at the medical school to their new location at Hoffheimer Hall. Movers carried boxes laden heavy with text books and the physician giants of IVF I had up until then only read about were picking up odds and ends from their recently departed offices. Howard and Georgeanna Jones or Drs. Howard and Georgeanna as they liked to be called looked to me on that auspicious day like someone's grandparents rather than the father and mother of IVF. I feared that I had come too late, that they were way past their prime and I would not be able to learn from them. It was after all 1985 and they had been leaders in infertility since the 1950's. Dr. Howard was forced into retirement from Johns Hopkins Hospital almost 7 years earlier after his 65th birthday.

They had planned to settle on the Maryland shore and spend time on their second love after fertility, sailing. Instead, an old friend of theirs from Johns Hopkins from the 1960's, Mason Andrews, helped found a new medical school in Norfolk, Virginia and now wanted their help to build the division of Reproductive Endocrinology, Infertility (REI). Eastern Virginia Medical School was new and barely known by anyone outside of Virginia at that time. Mason, a southern gentleman in his 60's, soft spoken with a sharp wit and former Mayor of Norfolk, was successful in talking them into spending a few more years teaching so they bought a cozy home on the Elizabeth River 10 minutes from the school.

The Joneses hadn't finished unpacking when the greatest fertility event of all time hit the news. Patrick Steptoe and Robert Edwards had succeeded in Great Britain with creating a new life through a process known as In Vitro Fertilization. The Joneses had worked with Professor Edwards years ago and were themselves well known in the field so it was natural that journalists came to their home to interview the erudite couple. Dr. Howard spoke about the genius of Professor Edwards and how he was not surprised that he had achieved success. Almost as an afterthought at the end of the interview, Dr. Jones was asked if IVF could be performed successfully in Norfolk. In Dr. Howard's pinpoint precision fashion and with his classic radio announcer voice, proclaimed that with sufficient funds they could create a successful IVF program in Norfolk. I have seen videotapes of Dr. Howard talking about this moment and it conjures up images of Babe Ruth promising to hit a homerun for the sick boy in the hospital then pointing to the fence just prior to him knocking one out of the park.

Well, the Joneses hit the homerun as predicted and by the time I arrived in 1985, Norfolk was the center of the IVF universe. Experts worldwide travelled to Norfolk to train and to teach. Prior to the Joneses entering the playing field of IVF, the world averaged one baby a year from IVF. Dr. Georgeanna introduced the concept of stimulating a woman's ovaries with gonadotropin hormones in order to produce multiple eggs, thereby increasing the odds of retrieving healthy mature eggs, getting them fertilized and creating embryos that had good pregnancy potential. Patients travelled from all over to have their IVF at Norfolk, where the success rate in 1985 was a world leading 15%.

I was excited beyond belief that this was my world now. I arrived early that first day of my fellowship dressed in a brand new shirt and tie eager to learn and impress. I managed to be accepted to this most competitive fellowship in part because I had been reading reproductive endocrinology for over 5 years. I went through my ob gyn residency with the intention of specializing in REI and IVF. In 1980 I began my training in REI mentored by Zev Rosenwaks, who convinced me that I could not possibly learn as much in any other residency as I would with him in Stony Brook. So, I joined Zev, who had trained with the Joneses at Johns Hopkins, and he helped me start a residency clinic in REI at Stony Brook where I trained until 1985. I spent those five years preparing for this moment in July 1985, to do my fellowship with Howard and Georgeanna Jones at the world famous Jones Institute in Norfolk, Virginia.

That first day, during office hours, I was following Dr, Georgeanna who was seeing her private patients. Training begins. The professor quizzed the neophyte student, me, "do I know about the two cell theory to the luteal phase?" I was dumbfounded. I had never come across such a concept in any of my reading. Little did I know, Dr. Georgeanna had a knowledge base and theories in reproductive endocrinology that few others could rival. She explained about the large cell and small cell and how the small cell is activated 10 days after ovulation by the pregnancy hormone, hcg. In its absence the large cell dies, progesterone decreases and a woman menstruates. In its presence the activated small cells continue to pump out progesterone and support the pregnancy. How exciting! I realized that I would spend every possible free moment talking reproductive endocrinology with Dr. Georgeanna. She knew all the REI secrets. She was the endocrinologist expert of the team. She was also the heart of Norfolk. She empathized with her patients and would go out of her way for them to help her patients achieve their dream, and that dream was to build their family. Dr. Howard was the surgeon, the geneticist and the spokesman in addition to being the leader. He was able to motivate and direct like a general leading his troops to battle. Everyone on his team was critical in his view to their ultimate success. He loved to say, "a chain is only as strong as its weakest link". He did what he could to ensure the integrity of each link. Despite his age, 72, Dr. Howard exercised regularly, was in excellent shape and in my mind was the original Macho Man. I remember observing him operate, not always delicate, but experienced in fertility surgery like few others. He was never intimidated and if the job called for raw muscle he was eager and willing to provide it himself.

I completed my two year fellowship in 1987, having learned an enormous amount of information and prepared to start my own IVF program. However, the Joneses asked me to stay on as an assistant professor, to help start an embryo cryopreservation program and direct the donor egg program. How could I refuse such an opportunity? I saw patients next door to Dr. Georgeanna and around the corner from Dr. Howard. Zev Rosenwaks was down the hall. I could present every patient to whomever I thought would know the most about my patient's problems. This became an even better learning experience than my fellowship. There were four of us in the IVF rotation, Zev Rosenwaks, myself, Suheil Muasher, a fellow who was two years ahead of me in training and Anibal Acosta, the Howard Jones of Argentina. Rosenwaks and Acosta were often lecturing so Suheil and I performed more of the IVF that year. It was an exciting time. We started performing retrievals transvaginally instead of laparoscopically. We were experimenting with lupron and pregnancy rates were exceeding 25%. I was doing my life's dream working in IVF; helping women in need of help with conception achieve their dream of making their family.

Times were changing. Successful IVF programs were springing up throughout the nation. It was the spring of 1988 when I returned home and started the first successful IVF program on Long Island dedicated to Howard and Georgeanna Jones who through their time, efforts and knowledge trained me and in so doing passed the baton of successful family building through the miracle of IVF. Today, we remember these giants of IVF who started it all. Mason Andrews and Dr. Georgeanna have since passed on. Dr. Howard, now in his 90's and how he describes it as late in the 9th inning is still occasionally involved in trying to make IVF more accessible to the public. They were erudite medical pioneers who are responsible for the greater than million babies who have been born through the technology that they helped create and promote. They were the original teachers of IVF who selflessly shared their knowledge with others so that they also may help their patients conceive. I am eternally thankful for the opportunities and training I received there from them, from Zev Rosenwaks, Suheil Muasher and from others at the Institute.

THE JOURNEY BEGINS

THE PREGNANCY TEST IS NEGATIVE AGAIN, WHAT DO I DO?

WOMEN confronted with a negative result from a pregnancy test are always disappointed and sometimes devastated. Many admit to becoming depressed and find it hard to associate with people and in places where there are pregnant women or babies. This gets extremely uncomfortable in social situations when a close friend or family member is enjoying that very thing that you are being denied. A negative test is a reminder of all those feelings of emptiness, sadness and grief over the void created by infertility.

We do not have control over these feelings and emotions. They affect our whole being and unchecked will continue until they have caused a complete state of depression. I am writing this article to arm you with a strategy to fight the potentially damaging effects that infertility threatens to do to you and your life.

First, upon seeing or hearing that gut wrenching news, breathe. Meditation, by controlling and focusing on one's breathing can help you gain control of your emotions and calm your body, slow down your heart rate and assist you on focusing rationally on the issues. This can be difficult to achieve on your own and it helps to share this battle with your partner or a special someone who can help you to calm down and regain control. Second, it is important to put this trauma into perspective. It doesn't always help to hear that someone else is suffering worse whether it is earthquake victims or cancer victims but knowledge that fertile couple's only conceive 20% of the time every month means that you are in good company with plenty of future moms and dads.

The third step is seeking help from a specialist, a reproductive endocrinologist (REI) who has 7 years of post graduate training with much of it spent on helping patients with the same problem you have. He will seek to establish a diagnosis and offer you an option of treatments. He will work with you to develop a plan based on your diagnosis, age, years of infertility, motivation as well your financial and emotional means to support the therapy.

If you are already under the care of a reproductive endocrinologist the first two steps regarding dealing with the negative pregnancy test are the same. The third step becomes developing a plan with your REI or evaluating your current plan.

It is important that you understand the odds of success per cycle for the current treatment regimen that you are on. You want to establish why it may not have worked this time. It is the REI's job to offer recommendations either for continuing the present course of therapy explaining the odds of success, cost and risks or for alternative more aggressive and successful treatments again offering his opinion regarding the success, costs and risks of the other therapies.

These therapies may be surgical, such as laparoscopy or hysteroscopy to remove endometriosis, scar tissue, repair fallopian tubes or remove fibroids. They may be medical such as including the using of ovulation inducing agents like clomid or gonadotropin injections, and may include intrauterine insemination (IUI) with or without medications. They may include minimal stimulation IVF or full stimulated IVF. Age, duration of infertility, your diagnosis and ovarian condition and financial and emotional means play a large role in determining this plan that the REI must make with your input.

It could be that there remain diagnostic tests, yet undone that may prove value in ascertaining the diagnosis and facilitate treatment. These include a hysteroscopy or hydrosonogram to evaluate the uterine cavity as well as the HSG, hysterosalpingogram to evaluate the patency of the fallopian tubes as well as the uterine cavity.

Complementary therapies offer additional success potential by improving the health and wellness of an individual and therefore her fertility as well. These therapies have been associated with improved pregnancy rates seen when used as an adjunct to assisted reproductive technologies. They include: Acupuncture, massage, nutrition, psychological mind and body programs, hypnotherapy, etc.

The negative pregnancy test can throw you off balance, out of your routine and depress you. I have offered a plan to take control and not just improve your mood and life but increase the likelihood that your next test will be a positive one.

WHAT ARE MY ODDS?

One of the first questions that most people ask is "what is my chance for success?" In 2002 about 28% of cycles in the United States in which women underwent IVF and embryo transfer with their own eggs resulted in the live birth of at least one infant. This rate has been improving slowly but steadily over the years. Patients should be aware, however, that some clinics define "success" as any positive pregnancy test or any pregnancy, even if miscarried or ectopic. These "successes" are irrelevant to patients desiring a baby. To put these figures into perspective, studies have shown that the rate of pregnancy in couples with proven fertility in the past is only about 20% per cycle. Therefore, although a figure of 28% may sound low, it is greater than the chance that a fertile couple will conceive in any given cycle.

Success varies with many factors. The age of the woman is the most important factor, when women are using their own eggs. Success rates decline as women age. In fact the diminishing success accelerates even more dramatically after about age 37. Part of this decline is due to a lower chance of getting pregnant from ART, and part is due to a higher risk of miscarriage with increasing age. There is, however, no evidence that the risk of birth defects or chromosome abnormalities (such as Down's syndrome) is any different with ART than with natural conception.

Success rates vary with the number of embryos transferred. However, transferring more embryos at one time not only increases the chance of success with that transfer, but will also increase the risk of a multiple pregnancy, which is much more complicated than a singleton pregnancy. The impact of the number of embryos that are transferred on success rates also varies with the age of the woman.

Pregnancy complications, such as premature birth and low birth weight, tend to be higher with ART pregnancies, primarily because of the much higher rate of multiple pregnancies. Nationally, in 2002-2003 about 30% of ART deliveries were twin deliveries, versus 1-2% of spontaneous pregnancies. The risk of pregnancy containing triplets or more was 6% in 2003 but dropped to 2% in 2007.

As women get older, the likelihood of a successful response to ovarian stimulation and progression to egg retrieval decreases. These cycles in older women that have progressed to egg retrieval are also slightly less likely to reach transfer. The percentage of cycles that progress from transfer to pregnancy significantly decreases as women get older. As women get older, cycles that have progressed to pregnancy are less likely to result in a live birth because the risk for miscarriage is greater. This age related decrease in success accelerates after age 35 and even more so after age 40. Overall, nationally, 37% of cycles started in 2003 among women younger than 35 resulted in live births. This percentage decreased to 30% among women 35–37 years of age, 20% among women 38–40, 11% among women 41–42, and 4% among women older than 42. The proportion of cycles that resulted in singleton live births is even lower for each age group.

The success rates vary in different programs in part because of quality, skill and experience but also based on the above factors of age, number of embryos transferred and patient population. Patients may also differ by diagnosis and intrinsic fertility which may relate to the number of eggs a patient may be able to stimulate reflected by their baseline FSH and antral follicle count as well as the genetics of their gametes. These differences make it nearly impossible to compare programs. Another factor often overlooked when considering one's odds of conceiving and having a healthy baby from an IVF procedure is the success with cryo-preserved embryos.

Thus, a program which may have a lower success rate with a fresh transfer but much higher success with a frozen embryo transfer will result in a better chance of conceiving with only a single IVF stimulation and retrieval. Success with frozen embryos transferred in a subsequent cycle also allows the program to transfer fewer embryos in the fresh cycle minimizing the chance for conceiving a riskier multiple pregnancy. It may be more revealing to examine a program's success with a combination of the fresh embryo transfer and frozen embryo transfers resulting from a single IVF stimulation and retrieval. For example, at East Coast Fertility, the combined number of fresh and frozen embryo transfers that resulted in live births for women under age 35 from January 1, 2002 through December 2007 was 394. The number of retrievals during that time was 656. The successful live birth rate combining the fresh and frozen pregnancies divided by the number of retrievals was 60.1%. The high frozen embryo transfer pregnancy rate allowed us to transfer fewer embryos resulting in only 3 sets of triplets created over this six year period of time. All three were the result of identical twinning with 100% implantation from transfers of two embryos.

What can I do to increase my odds?

Patients often ask if there are any additional procedures we can do in the lab that may improve the odds for conception. Assisted hatching is the oldest and most commonly added procedure aimed at improving an embryo's ability to implant. Embryos must break out or hatch from their shell that has enclosed them since fertilization prior to implanting into the uterine lining. This can be performed mechanically, chemically and most recently by utilizing a laser microscopically aimed at the zona pellucidum, the shell surrounding the embryo. Assisted hatching appears to benefit most those patients who are older than 38 years of age and those with thick zonae.

Recently a protein additive called "Embryo glue" was shown to improve implantation rates in some patients whose embryos were transferred in media containing the "Embryo glue". "Embryo Glue" contains a protein called hyaluronan which is associated with implantation and is thought to be largely responsible for improving pregnancy rates with IVF.

Embryo co-culture is the growth of developing embryos in the same Petri dish as another cell line. Programs utilize either the woman's endometrial cells obtained from a previous endometrial biopsy or cumulus cells obtained at the time of the egg retrieval from the same follicles aspirated as the eggs. Growth factors produced by these endometrial and cumulus cell lines diffuse to the developing embryo and are thought to aid in the growth and development of the embryo. The two cell lines have a dynamic relationship. The cumulus cells can supply deficient nutrients and remove toxins from the developing embryo further aiding the embryo's development. The cumulus cells also secrete hyaluronan thus aiding implantation.

WHERE DO YOU GO?

SART DATA- Birth Rates, Triplet Rates

Like any other investment you want to ensure that you are optimizing your upside potential. When considering your fertility investment your goal is a healthy baby. Multiple pregnancies present a higher risk to the fetus, especially when there are more than two present. It stands to reason that when doing your due diligence on potential IVF programs that you check their success rates. Understanding how to read these rates is not always a simple matter. In addition, programs that transfer high numbers of embryos may inflate their pregnancy and birth rates but have uncomfortably high rates of the potentially dangerous triplets. The most recent data on IVF programs' success rates may be obtained from the website of the IVF society, the Society of Assisted Reproductive Technology, found on www.SART.org. It is important to understand the source of the numerator and denominator in any rate that you are reviewing. Live birth rates are most useful since it is measuring the ultimate goal. However, they may be reported using varying denominators such as retrieval or embryo transfer. Personally, I think that since the stimulation and retrieval are the most expensive, stressful and risky parts of the process that this should serve as the most accurate measure of success and therefore be used in the denominator. Embryos transferred that were frozen in a prior cycle do not put a patient through the risk or stress of stimulation and retrieval and is much less costly. I prefer to measure the number of pregnancies and live births from fresh and frozen embryo transfer cycles per retrieval. If one is only reporting live birth rates from fresh cycles check their frozen embryo transfer rates and their triplet rates. I would rather see a lower live birth rate per retrieval from fresh transfers if the frozen embryo transfer rate is high and the triplet rate is low than a high live birth rate associated with dangerously high triplet rates.

Benefits and Disadvantages of large programs – How long is the wait for monitoring in the AM?

Many large programs have vast experience due to the high number of patients they have cared for. That experience may translate into providing you with the most state of the art care. The physicians and embryologists in these large programs may have more skill due to the higher number of procedures they perform.

But, be prepared to wait…and wait…and wait…Some of the larger programs process up to or even greater than 100 patients in the morning during which time they have an assembly line of blood drawers and ultrasonographers. It is rare that your physician will actually perform your ultrasound and see for him/herself how your follicles are progressing and be available for questions. Often in large programs, the physicians will rotate making the decisions on all the patients monitored that day as well as rotate performing the procedures on all patients undergoing retrievals and transfers. If it is important to you that your doctor manages your case and performs your procedures then make sure you choose a program where you will have that contact with your physician.

How is the Embryo Transfer Performed and who performs it?

Studies have demonstrated improved success rates when embryos are transferred at least 1 cm from the top of the uterine cavity. I presented my own research in abstracts on this in 1999 and 2000 at our national ASRM meeting. This can only be confirmed using ultrasound guidance. There are some cases where the transfer catheter curls on itself in the cervical canal. This may not be appreciated without ultrasound guidance confirming the presence of the catheter in the uterine cavity.

I have seen significantly higher pregnancy rates when utilizing a two step transfer technique with the Wallace catheter. An initial catheter is inserted into the canal with the hub accessible outside the vagina. The catheter with the embryos is then easily fed atraumatically through this hub and into the uterine cavity. We place a cervical suture to straighten the cervical canal and improve access to the uterus. The suture is essential to improving success in more difficult transfers. This technique combined with performing a trial transfer allows physicians to insert the transfer catheter without causing trauma or uterine contractions which might otherwise diminish a woman's chances of conceiving with her IVF cycle.

Even though many large programs have some very experienced personnel and physicians, others may not be so experienced. Do you know who is going to do your procedure? Is the physician performing your embryo transfer someone you have met before who knows and cares about you as a person? Has he/she put a catheter through you or your wife's cervix before? Does he/she have the same pregnancy rates as the rest of the program?

MEET THE DOCTOR

It is preferable for a husband to accompany his wife when she meets the doctor for the first time for several reasons. The two of you can compare notes as to what was said and whether this doctor and program seems to be a good match for you. It is common for patients to feel stressed when meeting the doctor and may not hear, understand or remember much of what is said. When you are there as a couple, it is easier to question when you do not understand and get a better appreciation and understanding of the presentation by the doctor and program. Do you and your wife connect with the doctor? Both of you should feel comfortable as this is the most important individual you will be relying on for your IVF process.

Doctors often communicate in their own medical language but sometimes may not realize that a patient doesn't understand. Your job is to make sure the doctor clarifies in language that both of you can understand. If he cannot make you understand that does not bode well for doing well in that program. Communication is essential to a successful IVF. There are many steps you and your wife must go through. If you miss something or do it wrong, it can make the difference between success and failure. One of the things you should assess on that first meeting is whether you will be able to follow directions presented by this office. If you have difficulties how easy is it to rectify before it is too late. Do you have a primary nurse responsible for you? Does the program have a patient advocate who you can turn to solve any problems you may be having? How accessible is your doctor? Now, with email available on phones, it is possible for my patients to have access to me 24/7. Patients can now have their questions answered by me as soon as it occurs to them.

The purpose of the initial consultation is mutual assessment and development of a plan. You should understand your options, your odds of success with these options and a proposed plan of action. The doctor assesses your medical situation, evaluates and makes recommendations. You assess the doctor and program. You evaluate the proposed plan and decide whether to follow it with this doctor.

CAUSES OF
INFERTILIY

HAVE YOU HAD A FERTILITY WORKUP?

I have received an enormous amount of email from patients over the years asking for information about how they should get started with their infertility workup. Apparently, they are women, men and couples who have experienced difficulty conceiving and now want some direction about how they should proceed. Building a family was something they had imagined their entire lives to be a natural progression--from student to career, getting married then having a family--and they're frustrated that their difficulty conceiving has affected their lives. For many—some of whom have never experienced a health problem-- it prevents them from appreciating or even doing anything else.

SEE AN RE FOR A FERTILITY WORKUP

My response to these emails has been to tell the patients to seek assistance from a reproductive endocrinologist, whose specialty and experience is in helping infertility patients conceive. A reproductive endocrinologist, who has two to three years of additional specialty fellowship training in infertility after completing an OB/GYN residency.

The RE will conduct a history and physical examination during your initial consultation. This exam typically includes a pelvic ultrasound of a woman's ovaries and uterus. He/she can tell if there are any uterine abnormalities that may affect implantation or pregnancy as well as assess ovarian activity and rule out cases of moderate or severe endometriosis.

Pelvic Inflammatory Disease

If he elicits a history of previous abdominal or pelvic surgery, a physician may suspect that scarring may have developed that typically interferes with fallopian tube transport of the egg to the sperm and the conceptus to the uterus. An infection that develops after a pregnancy may lead to pelvic adhesions affecting the tubes as well as scarring within the uterine cavity itself which can prevent implantation. Pelvic inflammatory disease, PID, can lead to tubal disease and may be associated with other sexually transmitted diseases including HPV, Herpes and especially Chlamydia.

Semen Analysis

The semen analysis is the simplest test to perform and will reveal a male factor in 50% of cases. A post coital test performed midcycle around the time of ovulation when the cervical mucus should be optimal can detect a male factor or cervical factor when few motile sperm are detected within hours of intercourse.

Hysterosalpingogram

A hysterosalpingogram, HSG, is a radiograph x-ray of the uterus and fallopian tubes after radio opaque contrast is injected vaginally through the cervix directly into the uterus. It can detect uterine abnormalities that can affect implantation and pregnancy as well as tubal patency. Unfortunately, this exam may be painful and in some patients with PID can result in serious infection. Some physicians will administer antibiotics prophylactically for this reason.

Hydrosonogram

A hydrosonogram is an ultrasound of the uterine cavity performed after injecting water vaginally through the cervix directly into the uterus. It can also detect uterine abnormalities and shares some of the risks seen with HSG but to a lesser extent and usually with less associated discomfort.

Hysteroscopy

A hysteroscopy is a surgical procedure in which a telescope is placed vaginally through the cervix directly into the uterus. The physician can visually inspect the cavity to detect uterine abnormalities. The risks of pain and infection are also seen with hysteroscopy.

Blood Tests

Blood tests may be run to identify if a patient is ovulating with adequate progesterone stimulation of the uterine lining. Day 3 E2, FSH and LH levels can give information regarding ovarian activity and ovulatory dysfunction. AntiMullerian Hormone (AMH) levels correlate with ovarian reserve. That is the number of eggs remaining in the ovaries. Hormones that can affect fertility such as thyroid and prolactin are also assessed to ensure that extraneous endocrine problems are not the cause of the infertility.

Laparoscopy

Laparoscopy is a surgical procedure in which a telescope is placed abdominally through the navel thereby allowing a physician to inspect the pelvic organs. He/she can identify endometriosis, cysts, adhesions, infection, fibroids etc. that may be causing the infertility. Unfortunately, only about 25% of cases in women who have a laparoscopy performed will conceive because of treatment performed at the time of the laparoscopy.

Workup Results and Treatment

Treatment can be directed at the cause such as surgery to correct adhesions or remove endometriosis, uterine polyps or fibroids. Treatment can also be independent of the cause but improve fertility nonetheless. Ovulation induction increases the number of eggs and therefore the likelihood that an egg will fertilize. Gonadotropin injections stimulate many more eggs to develop in a cycle than clomid fertility pills. IVF with minimal or full stimulation is the most successful treatment for any cause of infertility. The decision as to what treatment to undertake will depend on numerous factors including your age, duration of infertility, cause of infertility, cost of treatment and success of treatment as well as your insurance coverage for the treatment and your motivation to conceive and willingness to accept the risks associated with the treatment. Today, there is a highly successful treatment available for nearly all women.

ARE FIBROIDS AND POLYPS PREVENTING YOU FROM GETTING PREGNANT?

Fertility is dependent upon so many things!

First it must involve healthy gametes (eggs) capable of fertilizing and implanting in a uterus with a normal endometrial lining unimpeded by any uterine or endometrial pathology. Then, it requires sperm (in sufficient number) that are capable of swimming up through a cervix which is not inflamed and provides a mucous medium that promotes sperm motility. The eggs need to ovulate and be picked up by normal healthy fimbriated ends (finger like projections) of the fallopian tubes. The tubes need to be covered with normal micro hairs called cilia that help transport the egg one third of the way down the tube where one of the sperm will fertilize it.

The united egg and sperm (the "conceptus") then needs to undergo cell division, growth and development as it traverses the tube and makes its way to the uterine cavity by the embryo's fifth day of life at which point it is a blastocyst. The blastocyst hatches out of its shell ("zona pellucidum") and implants into the endometrial lining requiring adequate blood flow.

And you wonder why getting pregnant is so hard?

Now, on top of all that, occasionally, an intramural myoma (fibroid in the uterine muscle wall) may obstruct adequate blood flow to the endometrial lining. However, it is the submucosal myoma, inside the uterine cavity, that produces an IUD-like effect of irritating the uterine lining which can prevent implantation. Endometrial polyps (endometrial tissue protruding into the uterine cavity) may have a similar effect.

If your pregnancy is being hindered by these growths, you may need to have a **hydrosonogram**. A hydrosonogram is a procedure where your doctor or a radiologist injects water through your cervix into your uterus while performing a transvaginal ultrasound of your uterus. On the ultrasound, the water shows up as black against a white endometrial border. A defect in the smooth edges of the uterine cavity caused by an endometrial polyp or fibroid may be easily seen.

The hydrosonogram is performed by placing a thin tubular plastic catheter through the cervix into the uterine cavity. Water is injected using a syringe connected to a plastic tube. A patient may feel mild cramping, which is occasionally worse when she has fallopian tube disease or obstruction. Sometimes, at this point, a doctor will also use an embryo transfer catheter and perform an embryo transfer trial in anticipation of an in vitro fertilization (IVF) cycle.

Both polyps and fibroids in the uterine cavity can cause abnormal vaginal bleeding and occasionally cramping. These polyps and fibroids are almost always benign but they may need to be removed to render implantation. An endometrial polyp may be removed by a hysteroscopy, dilatation and curettage procedure. A hysteroscopy is performed vaginally, while a patient is asleep under anesthesia. A scope is placed through the cervix into the uterus in order to look inside the uterine cavity. This procedure can often be performed as an outpatient in an ambulatory or office based surgery unit. The risk of bleeding, infection or injury to the uterus is extremely rare.

Resection of a submucosal myoma is more difficult and is a longer procedure than the polypectomy. It too is performed hysteroscopically, without cutting. Sometimes, especially when the fibroid is large, it will take multiple procedures in order to remove the fibroid in its entirety. It will be necessary to repeat the hydrosonogram after the fibroid resection to make sure the cavity is satisfactory for implantation.

Are polyps or fibroids preventing you from getting pregnant?

Though the procedures I've described above are no picnic, failure to do them to remove endometrial polyps and submucosal myomata will not only prevent your pregnancy from occurring spontaneously, it will prevent implantation even with IVF!

HYDROSALPINX

A hydrosalpinx is a fallopian tube that is blocked at its distal end on the opposite side from the entrance to the uterine cavity. It may be diagnosed by a hysterosalpingogram or in severe cases by pelvic ultrasound. The hydrosalpinx is filled with inflammatory fluid and is most likely the end result of a pelvic infection. This inflammatory fluid can flow into the uterus and provide a hostile environment that will prevent implantation of an embryo. Research has shown that removing the hydrosalpinx (salpingectomy) or closing it off from the uterus such as with a tubal ligation significantly improves success with embryo transfer by preventing the flow of this inflammatory fluid into the uterus. Furthermore, transferred embryos will not uncommonly be pushed into the fallopian tubes after a uterine contraction. A healthy fallopian tube will sweep that embryo back into the uterine cavity with its cilia or microscopic hairs. A hydrosalpinx does not have healthy cilia so many of these embryos that find their way into the fallopian tube become trapped and may implant there resulting in a dangerous ectopic pregnancy that needs to be removed surgically if unable to destroy it medically.

A prophylactic salpingectomy or tubal ligation may be performed laparoscopically, using a tubular scope placed through the abdominal cavity to look inside the pelvis. Other instruments are placed through the lower abdominal wall and are used to remove the tube or close off the tube entrance to the uterus. Laparoscopy is performed under general anesthesia in the hospital.

Recently, the use of a contraceptive device, Essure, has been used to obstruct flow of the inflammatory fluid from the hydrosalpinx into the uterus. The Essure is a small coil that is inserted hysteroscopically through a woman's vagina without cutting into the fallopian tube. It takes 3 months to induce adequate scar closure of the tube and is as effective as a tubal ligation. A hysterosalpingogram is performed after the 3 month period to prove adequate damming of the flow of inflammatory fluid. This procedure may be performed in an office based surgical unit and is sometimes performed without anesthesia.

POLYCYSTIC OVARIAN DISEASE

Polycystic Ovary Syndrome (PCOS) is a condition in which a woman's hormones are out of balance. It can cause problems with your periods and make it difficult to get pregnant. PCOS may affect the way you look and can be associated with a variety of health problems including diabetes, hyperlipidemia and hypertension.

PCOS is the most common hormonal disorder of reproductive age women, occurring in over 7% of women at some point in their lifetime. It usually develops during the teen years. Treatment can assist women attempting to conceive, help control the symptoms and prevent long term health problems.

The most common cause of PCOS is glucose intolerance resulting in abnormally high insulin levels. If a woman does not respond normally to insulin, her blood sugar levels rise triggering the body to produce more insulin. The insulin stimulates your ovaries to produce male sex hormones called androgens. Testosterone is a common androgen and is often elevated in women with PCOS. These androgens block the development and maturation of a woman's ovarian follicles preventing ovulation resulting in irregular menses and infertility. Androgens may also trigger development of acne and extra facial and body hair. It will increase lipids in the blood. The elevated blood sugar from insulin resistance can develop into diabetes.

Symptoms may vary but the most common are acne, weight gain, extra hair on the face and body, thinning of hair on the scalp, irregular periods and infertility.

Ovaries develop numerous small follicles that look like cysts hence the name polycystic ovary syndrome. These cysts themselves are not harmful but in response to fertility treatment can result in a condition known as Hyperstimulation syndrome. Hyperstimulation syndrome involves ovarian swelling, fluid accumulating in the belly and occasionally around the lungs. A woman with Hyperstimulation syndrome may become dehydrated increasing her risk of developing blood clots. Becoming pregnant adds to the stimulation and exacerbates the condition leading many specialists to cancel cycles in which a woman is at high risk of developing Hyperstimulation. They may also prescribe aspirin to prevent clot formation.

These cysts may lead to many eggs maturing in response to fertility treatment also placing patients at a high risk of developing a high order multiple pregnancy. Due to this unique risk it may be advantageous to avoid aggressive stimulation of the ovaries unless the eggs are removed as part of an in vitro fertilization procedure.

A diagnosis of PCOS may be made by history and physical examination including an ultrasound of the ovaries. A glucose tolerance test is most useful to determine the presence of glucose intolerance and diabetes. Hormone assays will also be helpful in making a differential diagnosis.

Treatment starts with regular exercise and a diet including healthy foods with a controlled carbohydrate intake. This can help lower blood pressure and cholesterol and reduce the risk of diabetes. It can also help you lose weight if you need to.

Quitting smoking will help reduce androgen levels and reduce the risk for heart disease. Birth control pills help regulate periods and reduce excess facial hair and acne. Laser hair removal has also been used successfully to reduce excess hair.

A diabetes medicine called metformin can help control insulin and blood sugar levels. This can help lower androgen levels, regulate menstrual cycles and improve fertility. Fertility medications, in particular clomiphene are often needed in addition to metformin to get a woman to ovulate and will assist many women to conceive. The use of gonadotropin hormone injections without egg removal as performed as part of an IVF procedure may result in Hyperstimulation syndrome and/or multiple pregnancies and therefore one must be extremely cautious in its use. In vitro fertilization has been very successful and offers a means for a woman with PCOS to conceive without a significant risk for developing a multiple pregnancy especially when associated with a single embryo transfer. Since IVF is much more successful than insemination or intercourse with gonadotropin stimulation, IVF will reduce the number of potential exposures a patient must have to Hyperstimulation syndrome before conceiving.

It can be hard to deal with having PCOS. If you are feeling sad or depressed, it may help to talk to a counselor or to others who have the condition. Ask your doctor about support groups and for treatment that can help you with your symptoms. Remember, PCOS can be annoying, aggravating even depressing but it is fortunately a very treatable disorder.

ENDOMETRIOSIS

Background

The endometrium is the tissue that lines the inside of the uterine cavity. Endometriosis is a disease state in which some of this tissue has spread outside the uterus including the ovaries, or elsewhere in the abdominal cavity. Endometriosis causes pain in some women and can also cause infertility. Approximately 5-10% of all women have endometriosis. Many of these women are not infertile and many who are infertile do not have pain. Among patients who have infertility about 30% have endometriosis.

Making The Diagnosis

The only way to be sure whether a woman has endometriosis is to perform a surgical procedure called laparoscopy that allows your physician to look inside the abdominal cavity with a narrow tubular scope. He/she may be suspicious that you have endometriosis based on your history of very painful menstrual cycles, painful intercourse, etc., or based on your physical examination or ultrasound findings. On ultrasound, a cyst of endometriosis has a characteristic homogenous appearance showing echoes in the cyst that distinguish it from a normal ovarian follicle. Unlike the corpus luteum (ovulated follicle), its edges are round as opposed to collapsed and irregular in the corpus luteum and the cyst persists after a menses where corpora lutea will resolve each month.

Women with any stage of endometriosis (mild, moderate, or severe) can have severe lower abdominal and pelvic pain - or they might have no pain or symptoms whatsoever. Patients with mild endometriosis will not have a cyst and will have no physical findings on exam or ultrasound. It is thought that infertility caused by mild disease may be chemical in nature perhaps affecting sperm motility, fertilization, embryo development or even implantation perhaps mediated through an autoimmune response.

On the other had moderate and severe endometriosis are associated with ovarian cysts of endometriosis which contain old blood which turns brown and has the appearance of chocolate. These endometriomata (so called chocolate cysts) cause pelvic scarring and distortion of pelvic anatomy. The tubes can become damaged or blocked and the ovaries may become adherent to the uterus, bowel or pelvic side wall. Any of these anatomic distortions can result in infertility.

In some cases the tissue including the eggs in the ovaries can be damaged, resulting in diminished ovarian reserve and reduced egg quantity and quality.

Treatment of endometriosis

The treatment for endometriosis associated with infertility needs to be individualized for each woman. There are no easy answers, and treatment decisions depend on factors such as the severity of the disease and its location in the pelvis, the age of the woman, length of infertility, and the presence of pain or other symptoms. Some general issues regarding treatment are discussed here:

Treatment for mild endometriosis

Medical (drug) treatment can suppress endometriosis and relieve the associated pain in many women. Surgical removal of lesions by laparoscopy might also reduce the pain temporarily.

However, several well-controlled studies have shown that neither medical nor surgical treatment for mild endometriosis will improve pregnancy rates for infertile women as compared to expectant management (no treatment). For treatment of the infertility associated with mild to moderate endometriosis, ovulation induction with intrauterine insemination has a reasonable chance to result in pregnancy if no other infertility factors are present. If this is not effective after about 3-6 cycles (maximum), then in vitro fertilization would be recommended.

Treatment for severe endometriosis

Several studies have shown that medical treatment for severe endometriosis does not improve pregnancy rates for infertile women. Some studies have shown that surgical treatment of severe endometriosis does improve the chances for pregnancy as compared to no treatment. However, the pregnancy rates remain low after surgery perhaps no better than 2% per month.

Some physicians advocate medical suppression with a GnRH-agonist such as Lupron for up to 6 months after surgery for severe endometriosis before attempting conception. Although at least one published study found this to improve pregnancy rates as compared to surgery alone, other studies have shown it to be of no benefit. The older a patient is the more problematic post surgical treatment with lupron will be as it delays a woman's attempt to conceive until she is even older and less fertile due to aging.

Unfortunately, the infertility in women with severe endometriosis is often resistant to treatment with ovarian stimulation plus intrauterine insemination as the pelvic anatomy is much distorted. These women will often require in vitro fertilization in order to conceive. As endometriosis is a progressive destructive disorder that will lead to diminished ovarian reserve if left unchecked, it is vital to undergo a regular fertility screen annually and to consider moving up one's plans to start a family before one's ovaries become too egg depleted. When ready to conceive, it is recommended to proceed aggressively to the most effective and efficient therapy possible. Patients with endometriosis and infertility are unfortunately in a race to get pregnant before the endometriosis destroys too much ovarian tissue and achieving a pregnancy with one's own eggs becomes impossible.

ENDOMETRIOSIS AND YOUR INFERTILITY

I don't have to tell you that endometriosis can be a very painful illness and that it can cause infertility. It is often a reproductive life-long struggle in which tissue that normally lines the uterus migrates or implants into other parts of the body, most often in the pelvic lining and ovaries. Endometriosis may lead to pain and swelling and often times difficulty conceiving. You are not alone. Five to ten percent of all women have it. Though many of these women are not infertile, among patients who have infertility, about 30 percent have endometriosis.

Endometriosis can grow like a weed in a garden, irritating the local lining of the pelvic cavity and attaching itself to the ovaries and bowels. Scar tissue often forms where it grows, which can exacerbate the pain and increase the likelihood of infertility. The only way to be sure a woman has endometriosis is to perform a surgical procedure called laparoscopy which allows your physician to look inside the abdominal cavity with a narrow tubular scope. He may be suspicious that you have endometriosis based on your history of very painful menstrual cycles, painful intercourse, etc., or based on your physical examination or ultrasound findings. On an ultrasound, a cyst of endometriosis has a characteristic homogenous appearance showing echoes in the cyst that distinguish it from a normal ovarian follicle. Unlike the corpus luteum (ovulated follicle), its edges are round as opposed to collapsed and irregular in the corpus luteum and the cyst persists after a menses whereas corpora lutea will resolve each month.

Women with any stage of endometriosis (mild, moderate, or severe) can have severe lower abdominal and pelvic pain - or they might have no pain or symptoms whatsoever. Patients with mild endometriosis will not have a cyst and will have no physical findings on exam or ultrasound. It is thought that infertility caused by mild disease may be chemical in nature perhaps affecting sperm motility, fertilization, embryo development or even implantation perhaps mediated through an autoimmune response.

Moderate and severe endometriosis are, on the other hand, associated with ovarian cysts of endometriosis which contain old blood which turns brown and has the appearance of chocolate. These endometriomata (so called "chocolate cysts") cause pelvic scarring and distortion of pelvic anatomy. The tubes can become damaged or blocked and the ovaries may become adherent to the uterus, bowel or pelvic side wall. Any of these anatomic distortions can result in infertility. In some cases the tissue including the eggs in the ovaries can be damaged, resulting in diminished ovarian reserve and reduced egg quantity and quality.

The treatment for endometriosis associated with infertility needs to be individualized for each woman. Surgery often provides temporary relief and can improve fertility but rarely is successful in permanently eliminating the endometriosis which typically returns one to two years after resection.

There are no easy answers, and treatment decisions depend on factors such as the severity of the disease and its location in the pelvis, the woman's age, length of infertility, and the presence of pain or other symptoms.

Treatment for Mild Endometriosis

Medical (drug) treatment can suppress endometriosis and relieve the associated pain in many women. Surgical removal of lesions by laparoscopy might also reduce the pain temporarily.

However, several well-controlled studies have shown that neither medical nor surgical treatment for mild endometriosis will improve pregnancy rates for infertile women as compared to expectant management (no treatment). For treatment of infertility associated with mild to moderate endometriosis, ovulation induction with intrauterine insemination (IUI) has a reasonable chance to result in pregnancy if no other infertility factors are present. If this is not effective after about three - six cycles (maximum), then I would recommend proceeding with in vitro fertilization (IVF).

Treatment for Severe Endometriosis

Several studies have shown that medical treatment for severe endometriosis does not improve pregnancy rates for infertile women. Some studies have shown that surgical treatment of severe endometriosis does improve the chances for pregnancy as compared to no treatment. However, the pregnancy rates remain low after surgery, perhaps no better than two percent per month.

Some physicians advocate medical suppression with a GnRH-agonist such as Lupron for up to six months after surgery for severe endometriosis before attempting conception. Although at least one published study found this to improve pregnancy rates as compared to surgery alone, other studies have shown it to be of no benefit. The older a patient is the more problematic post surgical treatment with Lupron will be as it delays a woman's attempt to conceive until she is even older and less fertile due to aging.

Unfortunately, the infertility in women with severe endometriosis is often resistant to treatment with ovarian stimulation plus IUI as the pelvic anatomy is much distorted. These women will often require IVF in order to conceive.

Recommendations

As endometriosis is a progressive destructive disorder that will lead to diminished ovarian reserve if left unchecked, it is vital to undergo a regular fertility screen annually and to consider moving up your plans to start a family before your ovaries become too egg depleted. When ready to conceive, I recommend that you proceed aggressively to the most effective and efficient therapy possible.

Women with endometriosis and infertility are unfortunately in a race to get pregnant before the endometriosis destroys too much ovarian tissue and achieving a pregnancy with their own eggs becomes impossible. However, if you are proactive and do not significantly delay in aggressively proceeding with your family building, then I have every expectation that you will be successful in your efforts to become a mom.

WHAT DO YOU KNOW ABOUT YOUR FERTILITY?

David Kreiner, MD and Pamela Madsen

Women have a biological clock. Everyone knows that. The problem is that a lot of the information people think they know about their fertility and reproduction is not true. The blurring of fact, opinion, myth and misunderstanding makes for a treacherous misinformation landscape. The knowledge gap has claimed millions of victims, people who learned about their limited reproductive lifespan too late to help them have genetically linked offspring they always assumed would be theirs. Armed with essential and accurate information, you don't have to join their ranks.

What is still not understood across the board is the time line of the biological clock. And most women don't have a clue about their own.

So the big question is – what do you know about your fertility?

Well, if you're like most people, the answer is not as much as you might believe. Just to give you a little perspective, a spate of recent surveys reveals that the overwhelming majority of U.S. women:

- Don't understand the biological clock – the trajectory of reproductive capabilities from its peak in the early-to-mid-20s begins to decline, typically, around 27.
- Mistake overall good health for an indicator of fertility.

However wonderfully youthful and fit a 42-year-old might be, her eggs are operating on an independent and fixed timeline. The stark truth is women at that age are more likely than not to require medical intervention.

- Don't know that lifestyle factors—sleep, diet, exercise and environment, for instance – can have a profound effect on the ability to have a child.

Yet this basic information can make a critical difference in the life of every person who dreams of having a child. If you know about your body's reproductive lifecycle, you can take steps to protect and preserve your fertility and have the children you want– if and when you choose.

Marking Time: The Biological Clock and You

Each woman's oocytes (eggs) supply is finite. That means the body doesn't produce new ones. So the 7 million or so eggs each female is born with is all she's going to have. By the time the average girl hits puberty, only about 250,000-300,000 oocytes remain in her ovaries. With each menstrual cycle one egg is released, and an additional thousand eggs each month are lost through a process called artresia, the natural break-down of the eggs by the body. After ovulating an average of 400 times through her life, typically at around 50 years of age, the store of oocytes is tapped out. That's menopause.

Then there's the matter of oocyte aging. Eggs age along with the rest of the body. The older oocytes are more likely to have chromosomal abnormalities making them unlikely to become viable embryos. It's important to note that a fertilized egg with abnormal chromosomes is the single most common cause of miscarriage. As a general rule, women in their 20s have about a 20% chance of having a miscarriage each time she becomes pregnant, a woman in her 30's a 30% chance and a woman in her 40s about a 40% risk of miscarriage.

The bottom line is the older we get, the less likely we are to conceive and have a successful pregnancy. Fertility starts to decline when a woman is in her 20's but when she hits 35, it take a sharp downturn. At 40, fertility falls off even more dramatically.

Of course, some women in their late 30s and a few in their 40s conceive effortlessly, carry and deliver healthy babies. But the likelihood of that happening without medical intervention becomes more remote with each passing year. For women under 30, the estimated chance of becoming pregnant in any one cycle is between 20% and 30%. When women turn 40, that probability plummets to approximately 5%. Even more significant is that when a woman experiences difficulty conceiving in her 40's it is a far greater challenge to achieve a live birth using her own eggs even with the best medical technologies.

What Do You Know About Fertility Screening?

Statistics and general truths aside, every woman is unique. Given just how complicated it is to make a baby in the first place, understanding your own body's reproductive capability and the changes it might undergo from year to year is an invaluable planning tool.

Consider an annual fertility evaluation or screening

Simply put, the screening involves a few simple blood tests and an ultrasound to assess your ovarian function. These tests have been around for years, tried and true tools in the assessment of fertility.

We propose using these tests as a screen to prevent future infertility. We recommend that annual screening begin at 30 years of age or earlier if you have irregular menses, hot flashes, difficulty conceiveing after 6 months or a family history of early menopause or infertility.

Taken together with your individual and your family's medical histories, the screening helps establish where you are on your personal fertility curve. The first screening establishes your baseline, subsequent annual evaluations will flag changes in key hormone levels and mature follicle and egg production that could signal potential trouble. Mind you, any warning flares are just that and may mean nothing. But they could indicate that follow-up with your doctor, gynecologist or a reproductive specialist is warranted. And if there is problem, you're ahead of the game with the opportunity for early intervention and, where possible, corrective action.

Fertility screening can help identify women whose ovarian function is diminishing so they can get timely treatment. The fact is, some women in their 30's prematurely age from a reproductive perspective and their fertility may look more like that of a woman in her 40's.

What Does The Screen Involve?

The screening itself is fairly low-tech.

Part one consists of a blood test to check the levels of FSH (follicle stimulating hormone), estradiol and AMH (antimullerian hormone). The FSH and estradiol must be measured on the second or third day of your period. The granulosa cells of the ovarian follicles produce estradiol and AMH. The fewer the follicles there are in the ovaries the lower the AMH level. It will also mean that less estradiol is produced as well as a protein called inhibin. Both inhibin and estradiol decrease FSH production. The lower the inhibin and estradiol the higher the FSH as is seen in diminished ovarian reserve. The higher the estradiol or inhibin levels are then the lower the FSH. Estradiol may be elevated especially in the presence of an ovarian cyst even with failing ovaries that are only able to produce minimal inhibin. However, the high estradiol reduces the FSH to deceptively normal appearing levels. If not for the cyst generating excess estradiol, the FSH would be high in failing ovaries due to low inhibin production. This is why it is important to get an estradiol level at the same time as the FSH and early in the cycle when it is likely that the estradiol level is low in order to get an accurate reading of FSH.

Part two is a vaginal ultrasound to count the number of antral follicles in both ovaries. Antral follicles are a good indicator of the reserve of eggs remaining in the ovary. In general, fertility specialists like to see at least a total of eight antral follicles for the two ovaries. Between nine and twelve might be considered a borderline antral follicle count.

As you start to screen annually for your fertility, what you and your doctor are looking for is a dramatic shift in values from one year to the next.

What Does The Screen Indicate?

A positive screen showing evidence of potentially diminishing fertility is an alarm that should produce a call to action. When a woman is aware that she may be running out of time to reproduce she can take the family-planning reins and make informed decisions. The goal of fertility screening is to help you and every woman of childbearing years make the choices that can help protect and optimize your fertility.

Although none of these tests is in of and of themselves an absolute predictor of your ability to get pregnant, when one or more come back in the abnormal range, it is highly suggestive of ovarian compromise. It deserves further scrutiny. That's when it makes sense to have a discussion with your gynecologist or fertility specialist. Bear in mind, the "normal" range is quite broad. But when an "abnormal" flare goes off, you want to check it out.

It's important to remember that fertility is more than your ovaries. If you have risk factors for blocked fallopian tubes such as a history of previous pelvic infection, or if your partner has potentially abnormal sperm, then other tests are in order. And if, for example you do have blocked tubes, it's better to have them corrected sooner rather than later when the becoming pregnant is an urgent matter.

Fertility Preservation: The Egg Freezing Revolution and The Biological Clock

As so many women discovered late in life, procreation is a far more delicate and complicated process than most of us ever suspect. After all we spend so much time trying to avoid pregnancy, it never occurs to us that we may not be able to when we want.

So what do you do if you are in the midst of getting your degree or your career is on an upward trend that you don't want to derail? Until recently, the options were few and unreliable.

But the world of reproductive medicine is on the fast track to breakthroughs in egg freezing which is giving young women the opportunity to put the best of their oocytes into a safe deep freeze until they're ready to use them.

Some IVF Centers claim that they are ready to provide state of the art egg freezing right now to women with hundreds of healthy babies already born. Others, like East Coast Fertility, are in the midst of doing studies and offering discounts to patients who want to be a part of the Egg Freezing Studies.

With careful attention to your fertility through a program of annual fertility screening, early intervention with fertility treatment or egg freezing, we can eliminate most cases of infertility due to aging and diminishing ovarian reserve.

SPERM MEETS EGG – WHY DOESN'T IT WORK EVERY TIME?

Why me? My wife never had an infection, surgery or any other problem? I have no difficulty ejaculating and there's plenty to work with so why can my friends, neighbors and coworkers get pregnant and we can't?

I hear these questions daily and appreciate the frustrations, anger and stress felt by my patients expressing these feelings through such questions. There are many reasons why couples do not conceive. An infertility workup will identify some of these. A semen analysis will pick up a male factor in 50-60% of cases and in more than half of these cases the male has the only problem. A hysterosalpingogram will locate tubal disease in about 20% of cases. Another 20-25% of women do not ovulate or ovulate dysfunctionally preventing conception.

Even when a semen analysis is normal it is possible that a post coital test may identify that the problem is that the sperm is not reaching the egg. It may not be able to swim up the cervical canal into the womb and up the tubes where it should normally find an egg to fertilize. When these tests are normal a laparoscopy may be performed to identify the 20-25% of infertile women with endometriosis. However, even when the infertility workup is normal and there is no test that logically explains the lack of success in achieving a pregnancy; an IVF procedure may both identify the cause as failure of the egg to fertilize and treat it successfully by injecting sperm microscopically into the egg by a procedure called Intracytoplasmic Sperm Injection or ICSI.

What causes male factor infertility?

There are several potential causes of male factor infertility. Hormonal causes can be caused because of problems at the hypothalamic-pituitary level or at the testicular level. Normally, the hypothalamus regulates pituitary production of Follicle Stimulating Hormone (FSH) and Luteinizing Hormone (LH). FSH and LH drive the testis to produce sperm and testosterone. Deficiency of FSH or LH can lead to lack of ability to drive the testicular production of sperm and testosterone just as lack of gas will prevent a car from being able to run. Today, the most common reason for a man to have FSH and LH production shut off is from his use of anabolic steroids such as testosterone, hcg (human chorionic gonadotropin) and clomiphene (clomid). These all may provide negative feedback on the pituitary turning off FSH and LH production. One can also see elevated testosterone shutting down the testis with congenital adrenal hyperplasia and adrenal tumors.

Pituitary tumors, infarction, surgery, radiation and infiltrative processes can also diminish FSH and LH production. In the presence of low FSH and LH it may be useful to check for elevated prolactin levels to rule out a pituitary prolactinoma and obtain an MRI to check for other tumors or pituitary pathology.

Isolated deficiency of LH and FSH can occur (Kallmann's syndrome) and lead to diminished testis (hypogonadism). This occurs in 1 in 10,000 men. Less common defects are seen in hypothalamic stimulation of the pituitary and are usually associated with other congenital findings.

Abnormal thyroid and glucocorticoid (prednisone) excess can result in decreased spermatogenesis through effects on the hypothalamus and LH production or conversion of androgens (male hormone) to estrogens.

Testicular causes include the presence of tumor, chromosomal abnormalities, congenital absence of germ cells, drugs and radiation that are toxic to the testes, undescended testes and varicocoele.

Ten per cent of males with a sperm count fewer than 10 million and 20% of men with azospermia have a chromosomal abnormality. Kleinfelter's syndrome is a genetic disorder due to the presence of an extra x chromosome in the male. This occurs in 1 out of 500 males and is often seen in the mosaic form where some cells are 46 xy and some are 47 xxy. The testes tend to be small and these men have delayed sexual maturation, azospermia and gynecomastia (enlarged male breasts). There has been some success with ICSI of biopsied immature sperm cells.

Sertoli-cell only syndrome or germinal cell aphasia may have several causes including congenital absence of the germ cells, genetic defects or androgen resistance. Testicular biopsy shows complete absence of germinal elements. Men are azospermic yet virilize normally. Testes may have normal consistency but be slightly smaller in size. Testosterone and LH levels are normal but FSH is usually elevated. Men with testicular failure secondary to mumps, cryptorchidism or radiation/chemotherapy damage have smaller testes with a non uniform histologic pattern. The testes may have severe sclerosis and hyalinization. There is no treatment for this form of azospermia.

Gonadotoxic drugs like chemotherapy or radiation can affect the germinal epithelium because it is a rapidly dividing tissue and is susceptible to the interference imposed by these toxins on cell division. At radiation exposure below 600 rads, germ cell damage is reversible. Recovered spermatogenesis may take up to 2-3 years even when exposed to low doses of radiation. Elevated FSH levels reflect the impaired spermatogenesis and return to normal once the testes recover.

Orchitis occurs in 15-25% of males who contract mumps which is unilateral in 90% of cases. Testicular atrophy may take years to develop. At least two thirds of men with bilateral orchitis remain infertile for life.

Trauma either through accident or torsion of a testis is a relatively common cause of subsequent atrophy with potential diminished fertility.

Medical conditions such as renal failure, cirrhosis of the liver and sickle cell disease can all lead to low testosterone levels and decreased spermatogenesis.

Cryptorchidism occurs in 1 in 12 males. The undescended testis becomes abnormal after age 2. Even when unilateral, cryptorchid patients have reduced fertility potential.

The varicocoele is the most common finding in infertile men. It is the result of backflow of blood due to incompetent valves in the spermatic veins. 90% occur on the left and is found in 20% of males, 40% of the infertile population.

Fifty per cent of men with varicocoeles are fertile. It is thought that a varicocoele can cause infertility by elevating the temperature of the testis. Varicocoelectomies however are not universally helpful and remain somewhat controversial for many cases of infertility.

Unfortunately, at least 25-40% of infertile men have idiopathic infertility for which no cause may be identified.

Other causes of azospermia include congenital absence of the vas deferens or obstruction secondary to infection or surgery. These cases may be amenable to surgical reconstruction and/or ICSI with epididymal aspiration or testicular biopsy to obtain sperm. These are the most successful cases of ICSI associated with azospermia.

Sperm antibodies may be a relative cause of infertility in about 3-7% of cases. Treatment has been successful with intrauterine insemination and with ICSI.

Infections can affect sperm motility secondary to e coli, Chlamydia, mycoplasma, ureaplasma and trichomonas. Culture and treatment for asymptomatic infertile males remains controversial.

Sexual dysfunction is a presenting cause of male infertility in about 20% of cases. Decreased sexual drive, erectile dysfunction, premature ejaculation and failure of intromission are all potentially correctable causes of infertility.

Treatment of Male Infertility

Treatment depends on diagnosis. In cases where the FSH and LH are low with a normal head MRI, clomiphene may be of benefit. Clomiphene citrate (Clomid or Serophene) is one of the most widely used drugs in male infertility. It is a weak anti-estrogen that interferes with the normal feedback of circulating estrogens and results in an increase in GnRH that stimulates gonadotropin secretion. The resulting elevation in LH and FSH increases intratesticular testosterone levels and in theory should improve spermatogenesis. Gonadotropin therapy may be used if clomiphene is unsuccessful in the face of low FSH and LH.

If a pituitary tumor is found, surgery or medications to lower prolactin may restore spermatogenesis to normal.

An obstructed vas may be microsurgically reconstructed. Surgery may also be performed in the presence of a varicocoele.

Intrauterine insemination may improve delivery of sperm to an egg or in the absence of any sperm; artificial insemination with donor sperm is often successful.

Intracytoplasmic sperm injection into the egg in an IVF procedure is highly successful when sperm may be obtained through the ejaculate and even through testicular biopsy. When normal mature sperm are rare such as in testicular failure, associated with elevated FSH, ICSI is much less likely to result in fertilization and pregnancy. Immature sperm cells rarely can result in a healthy pregnancy.

Naturopathic Treatment

Naturopathic treatment for male infertility focuses on improving sperm quantity, sperm quality, and overall male reproductive health. There have been reports that sperm counts have fallen almost 50% since the 1930s. Although some dispute these findings, it is generally accepted that sperm counts are declining. The cause may be environmental and dietary and lifestyle changes may interfere with men's sperm production. If this is so, improving diet and making healthy lifestyle choices should positively impact male reproductive health.

Nutrition

The importance of a healthy diet cannot be overstated. To function properly, the reproductive system requires the proper vitamins and minerals. Nutritional deficiencies can impair hormone function, inhibit sperm production, and contribute to the production of abnormal sperm

- Eat a natural foods diet that focuses on fresh vegetables, fruits, whole grains, fish, poultry, legumes, nuts, and seeds.
- Drink 50% of body weight in ounces of water daily (e.g., a 150 lb man would drink 75 oz of water).
- Eliminate processed and refined foods (e.g., white flour), junk food, sugars, alcohol, and caffeine.
- Avoid saturated fats and hydrogenated oils (e.g., margarine); use olive oil.
- Pumpkin seeds are naturally high in zinc and essential fatty acids which are vital to healthy functioning of the male reproductive system. Eat pumpkin seeds to help maintain a healthy reproductive system.

Supplements

The following supplements may increase sperm count and/or motility. Allow 3-4 months for the supplements to work. The following is a list of supplements with their supposed benefit.

- Arginine - Take 4 gr daily. It is required to produce sperm. If the sperm count is below 10 million per ml, arginine probably will not provide any benefit.
- Coenzyme Q10 - Take 10 mg daily. Co Q10 may increase sperm count and motility.
- Flaxseed oil - Take 1 tbsp daily. Flaxseed is a source of essential fatty acids.
- L-carnitine - Take 3-4 grams daily. It is required for normal sperm function.
- Multivitamin-mineral - Buy a high-quality product and take one serving size (differs from brand to brand).
- Selenium - Take 200 mcg daily. Selenium may improve sperm motility.
- Vitamin B-12 - Take 1000 mcg daily. A B-12 deficiency reduces sperm motility and sperm count. Even if no deficiency exists, B-12 supplementation may help men with a sperm

count of less than 20 million per milliliter or a motility rate of less than 50%

- Vitamin C - Take 500 mg 2 times daily. Vit C is an antioxidant.
- Vitamin E - Take 400 IUs 2 times daily. Is an antioxidant and may improve sperms' ability to impregnate.
- Zinc - Take 30 mg 2 times daily. Zinc is required for a healthy male reproductive system and sperm production.

Herbal Medicine

Herbal remedies usually do not have side effects when used appropriately and at suggested doses. Occasionally, an herb at the prescribed dose causes stomach upset or headache. This may reflect the purity of the preparation or added ingredients, such as synthetic binders or fillers. For this reason, it is recommended that only high-quality products be used. As with all medications, more is not better and overdosing can lead to serious illness and death.

The following herbs may be used to treat male infertility:

- Ginseng (Panax ginseng) - Known as a male tonic (an agent that improves general health) and used to increase testosterone levels and sperm count. Siberian ginseng (Eleutherococcus senticosus) may also be used.
- Astragalus (Astragalus membranaceus) – May increase sperm motility.
- Sarsaparilla (>Smilax spp.) - Known as a male (and female) tonic.
- Saw palmetto (Serenoa repens) - Used for overall male reproductive health.

Other Recommendations:

Avoid alcohol. Alcohol consumption is associated with an increased number of defective sperm.

- Consider acupuncture.
- Do not smoke, or quit smoking. There is an association between smoking and low sperm count, poor sperm motility, and abnormal sperm.
- Proxeed - is a new nutritional supplement that may improve sperm health and fertility rates. The ingredients include L-carnitine and acetylcarnitine, two vitamin-like substances synthesized naturally by the body. These chemicals are involved in cellular metabolism and are found in semen at a rate that is proportionate to the amount of healthy sperm. Proxeed is purported to improve sperm count, concentration, and motility when taken orally for about 2 months. It is reported that approximately 30% of couples using it conceive. It is available without a prescription, although couples considering it should consult their physician.

TREATMENT OF INFERTILITY

TRYING TO CONCEIVE
WITH CLOMID THERAPY

IT has become commonplace for women who have been frustrated with repeated unsuccessful attempts to conceive naturally on their own to see their gynecologist who often times will try clomid therapy on them. Clomid, the traditional brand name for clomiphene citrate, is a competitive inhibitor of estrogen. It stimulates the pituitary gland to produce follicle stimulating hormone (FSH) which in turn will stimulate the ovaries to mature follicle(s) containing eggs. Estrogen normally has a negative feedback effect on the pituitary and is blocked by clomid leading to pituitary FSH production and ovarian stimulation.

Infertility patients, as defined by one year of unprotected intercourse without a resulting pregnancy, have a 2-5% pregnancy rate each month trying on their own without treatment. For women over 35, infertility is defined by six months of unprotected intercourse. Clomid therapy increases a couple's fertility by increasing the number of eggs matured in a cycle and by producing a healthier egg and follicle. The pregnancy rate with clomid therapy alone is approximately 10% per cycle and 12-15%. when combined with intrauterine insemination. Women who are unable to ovulate on their on experience a 20% pregnancy rate per cycle with clomid, the equivalent to that of a fertile couple trying on their own.

Those women who are likely to conceive with clomid usually do so in the first three months of therapy with very few conceiving after six months. As clomid has an antiestrogen effect, the cervical mucus and endometrial lining may be adversely affected. Cervical mucus is normally produced just prior to ovulation and may be noticed as a stringy egg white like discharge unique to the middle of a woman's cycle just prior to and during ovulation. It provides the perfect environment for the sperm to swim through to gain access to a woman's reproductive tract and find her egg. Unfortunately, clomid may thin out her cervical mucus preventing the sperm's entrance into her womb. Intrauterine insemination overcomes this issue through bypassing the cervical barrier and depositing the sperm directly into the uterus.

However, when the uterine lining or endometrium is affected by the antiestrogenic properties of clomid, an egg may be fertilized but implantation is unsuccessful due to the lack of secretory gland development in the uterus. The lining does not thicken as it normally would during the cycle. Attempts to overcome this problem with estrogen therapy are rarely successful.

Many women who take clomid experience no side effects. Others have complained of headache, mood changes, spots in front of their eyes, blurry vision, hot flashes and occasional cyst development that normally resolves on its own. Most of these effects last no longer than the five or seven days that you take the clomid and have no permanent side effect. The incidence of twins is 8-10% with a 1% risk of triplet development.

Yet, another deterrent to clomid use was a study performed years ago that suggested that women who used clomid for more than twelve cycles developed an increased incidence of ovarian tumors. It is therefore recommended by the American Society of Reproductive Medicine as well as the manufacturer of clomiphene that clomid be used for no more than six months after which it is recommended by both groups that patients proceed with treatment including gonadotropins (injectable hormones containing FSH and LH) to stimulate the ovaries in combination with intrauterine insemination or in vitro fertilization.

For patients who fail to ovulate on their own, clomid is successful in achieving a pregnancy in nearly 70% of cases. All other patients average close to a 50% pregnancy rate if they attempt six cycles with clomid especially when combined with intrauterine insemination. After six months the success is less than 5% per month. In vitro fertilization is a successful alternative therapy when other pelvic factors such as tubal disease, tubal ligation, adhesions or scar tissue and endometriosis exist or there is a deficient number, volume or motility of sperm. Success rates with IVF are age, exam and history dependent. The average pregnancy rate with a single fresh IVF cycle is greater than 50%. For women under 35, the pregnancy rate for women after a single stimulation and retrieval is greater than 70% with a greater than 60% live birth rate at East Coast Fertility. Young patients sometimes choose a minimal stimulation IVF or MicroIVF as an alternative to clomid/IUI cycles as a more successful and cost effective option as many of these patients experience a 40% pregnancy rate per retrieval at a cost today of $3900. Today, with all these options available to our patients, a woman desiring to build her family will usually succeed in becoming a mother.

INTRAUTERINE INSEMINATION (IUI)

Intrauterine insemination (IUI) is the least complex of the assisted reproductive technologies (ART) and is often tried as a first treatment in uncomplicated cases of infertility. IUI involves preparing sperm in the lab and delivering the washed and more motile sperm in a highly concentrated solution which is placed either directly into the cervix (intra-cervical insemination) or into the uterus (IUI). The standard procedure practiced in most reproductive endocrinology offices is IUI.

IUI can be performed with sperm from the male partner or a donor, and is often combined with ovulation induction by hormone therapy. It is useful treatment for women with open fallopian tubes and a normal uterine cavity and in cases where the man has a borderline low sperm count, volume or motility. It is also very useful as an adjunct to treating ovulation disorders by depositing optimized sperm when the egg is ovulating and ready for fertilization.

The Procedure

The IUI procedure involves monitoring of the woman's cycle with an ovulation predictor kit or hormone assays and pelvic ultrasounds to determine the timing of ovulation. Fertility drugs may also be taken in advance to increase the number of eggs released. At the time of ovulation, the man produces a semen specimen that is prepared in the laboratory resulting in a higher concentration and more motile form than his ejaculate. The semen specimen must be prepared or washed prior to being injected into the uterus because unwashed semen has chemicals that can cause extremely painful uterine cramping. The sperm are then placed in the uterus without anesthesia using a long thin catheter that is passed through the cervix directly into the uterus. This procedure takes place in the office exam room.

Success Rates

Success rates for IUI are based on the age of the woman, quality of sperm and the reason for infertility. The pregnancy rates per cycle were 7 percent for intrauterine insemination (IUI) alone and 10 percent to 17 percent per cycle for IUI combined with ovulation induction. Clomiphene (Clomid), a fertility pill that increases the pituitary FSH stimulation of the ovaries, is often used to increase the quantity and quality of eggs produced. It may cause side effects such as hot flashes, mood changes, blurry vision, and headache and cyst formation as well as increase the incidence of twins to 10% and triplets to 1%. It is not very effective after 3-6 cycles and has been cited as a possible cause of ovarian tumors when used more than 12 cycles.

Gonadotropins also may be used with IUI to increase the quantity and quality of eggs produced. It is far more effective and risky. There is a 3% risk of developing hyperstimulation syndrome, whereby the ovaries enlarge, fluid accumulates in the belly and can push up on the lungs causing difficulty with breathing. It may also cause dehydration increasing the risk of developing a blood clot.

Depending on diagnosis, physicians commonly suggest IUI as a reasonable first option for many women especially if they have insurance coverage for it. However, in cases where patients do not have insurance coverage for IUI, a safer and more cost effective treatment alternative is the minimal stimulation IVF or MicroIVF. It is approximately the same cost as IUI with gonadotropins but at least twice as effective. It does not put the patient at risk of developing hyperstimulation syndrome and the risk of a multiple pregnancy is far less.

MICROIVF

MicroIVF, also known as MiniIVF and minimal stimulation is an IVF procedure whereby a patient's ovaries are stimulated with oral medications (clomid) usually with a minimal amount of injectable gonadotropins. The process then proceeds in identical fashion to conventional IVF with egg retrieval, fertilization, embryo culture and ultrasound guided embryo transfer. This new protocol cuts down on costs and diminishes the risks of multiple births and hyperstimulation syndrome.

Young, healthy patients and patients with many follicles such as those with polycystic ovarian syndrome have the best response to the minimal stimulation typically producing multiple high quality embryos and allowing for cryopreservation of embryos available for a potential additional transfer in the future. When combined with East Coast Fertility's Single Embryo Transfer Program, the cryopreservation, embryo storage and future frozen embryo transfers are free.

As an alternative to intrauterine insemination, patients can triple their success and lower their risk at similar costs. Of course patients with pelvic adhesions/scarring, blocked fallopian tubes, endometriosis and severe male factor have an even lower or no chance of success with intrauterine insemination but yet their probability of success with MicroIVF is as good as that of any other patient.

The fee at East Coast Fertility for MicroIVF is currently $3900 but an additional $1000 fee is added if patients require ICSI to facilitate fertilization and/or $550 if anesthesia is requested. An IUI with hormone injections ranges from $3500 to $4500 including medication. The medication cost for MicroIVF is not much more than $100. Furthermore, one need not worry with MicroIVF that all the eggs ovulated may fertilize and implant as could happen with intrauterine insemination. The risk of high order multiple pregnancies that one faces with intrauterine insemination is eliminated with MicroIVF. You control how many embryos to transfer and therefore implant with IVF.

There is a risk of hyperstimulation syndrome associated with hormone injections that is essentially eliminated with MicroIVF. This condition can result in enlarged ovaries, abdominal swelling and bloating, fluid that can push up on the lungs causing difficulty with breathing. Patients can develop dehydration that can place them at risk of developing a blood clot. This is not a concern with the minimal stimulation. However, it is a significant risk with gonadotropins when used with intrauterine insemination.

In summary, MicroIVF, especially as an alternative to intrauterine insemination, offers a low cost, safer and more efficient means to build a family.

IN VITRO FERTILIZATION AND EMBRYO CULTURE

- Sperm and eggs are placed together in specialized conditions (culture media, controlled temperature, humidity and light) in hopes of fertilization.
- Culture medium is designed to permit normal fertilization and early embryo development.
- Embryo development in the lab helps distinguish embryos with more potential from those with less or none.

After eggs are retrieved, they are transferred to the embryology laboratory where they are kept in conditions that support their needs and growth. The embryos are placed in small dishes or tubes containing "culture medium," which is special fluid developed to support development of the embryos made to resemble that found in the fallopian tube or uterus. The dishes containing the embryos are then placed into incubators, which control the temperature and atmospheric gasses the embryos experience.

A few hours after the eggs are retrieved, sperm are placed in the culture medium with the eggs, or individual sperm are injected into each mature egg in a technique called Intracytoplasmic Sperm Injection (ICSI) (see below). The eggs are then returned to the incubator, where they remain overnight while going through fertilization.

The following day after the eggs have been inseminated or injected with a single sperm (ICSI), they are examined for signs that the process of fertilization is successful. At this stage, normal fertilization is confirmed by the still single cell having 2 pronuclei; the zygote. Two days after insemination or ICSI, normal embryos have divided into about 4 cells. Three days after insemination or ICSI, normally developing embryos contain about 8 cells. Five days after insemination or ICSI, normally developing embryos have developed to the blastocyst stage, which is typified by an embryo that now has 80 or more cells, an inner fluid-filled cavity, and a small cluster of cells called the inner cell mass.

It is important to note that since many eggs and embryos are abnormal, it is expected that not all eggs will fertilize and not all embryos will divide at a normal rate. The chance that a developing embryo will produce a pregnancy is related to whether its development in the lab is normal, but this correlation is not perfect. This means that not all embryos developing at the normal rate are in fact also genetically normal, and not all poorly developing embryos are genetically abnormal. Nonetheless, their visual appearance is the most common and useful guide in the selection of the best embryo(s) for transfer.

In spite of reasonable precautions, any of the following may occur in the lab that would prevent the establishment of a pregnancy:

- Fertilization of the egg(s) may fail to occur.
- One or more eggs may be fertilized abnormally resulting in an abnormal number of chromosomes in the embryo; these abnormal embryos will not be transferred.
- The fertilized eggs may degenerate before dividing into embryos, or adequate embryonic development may fail to occur.
- Bacterial contamination or a laboratory accident may result in loss or damage to some or all of the eggs or embryos.
- Laboratory equipment may fail, and/or extended power losses can occur which could lead to the destruction of eggs, sperm and embryos.
- Other unforeseen circumstances may prevent any step of the

procedure to be performed or prevent the establishment of a pregnancy.

- Hurricanes, floods, or other 'acts of God' (including bombings or other terrorist acts) could destroy the laboratory or its contents, including any sperm, eggs, or embryos being stored there.

Quality control in the lab is extremely important. Sometimes immature or unfertilized eggs, sperm or abnormal embryos (abnormally fertilized eggs or embryos whose lack of development indicates they are not of sufficient quality to be transferred) that would normally be discarded can be used for quality control.

MEDICATIONS FOR
IVF TREATMENT

- The success of IVF largely depends on growing multiple eggs at the same time.
- Injections of the natural hormones FSH and/or LH (gonadotropins) that are normally involved in ovulation every month are used for this purpose
- Additional medications are used to prevent premature ovulation

Gonadotropins, or injectable "fertility drugs" (Follistim®, Gonal-F®, Bravelle®,

- An overly vigorous ovarian response can occur, or conversely an inadequate response

Medications may include the following (not a complete list): **Menopur®):** These natural hormones stimulate the ovary in hopes of inducing the simultaneous growth of several oocytes (eggs) over the span of 8 or more days. All injectable fertility drugs have FSH (follicle stimulating hormone), a hormone that will stimulate the growth of your ovarian follicles (which contain the eggs). Some of them also contain LH (luteinizing hormone) or LH like activity. LH is a hormone that may work with FSH to increase the production of estrogen and growth of the follicles. Luveris®, recombinant LH, can also be given as a separate injection in addition to FSH or alternatively, low-dose hCG can be used. These medications are given by subcutaneous or intramuscular injection. Proper dosage of these drugs and the timing of egg recovery require monitoring of the ovarian response, usually by way of blood hormone tests and transvaginal follicular ultrasound examinations during the ovarian stimulation.

As with all injectable medications, bruising, redness, swelling, or discomfort can occur at the injection site. Rarely, there can be an allergic reaction to these drugs. The intent of giving these medications is to mature multiple follicles, and many women experience some bloating and minor discomfort as the follicles grow and the ovaries become temporarily enlarged. Up to 2.0 % of women will develop Ovarian Hyperstimulation Syndrome (OHSS).

Other risks and side effects of gonadotropins include, but are not limited to, fatigue, headaches, weight gain, mood swings, nausea, and clots in blood vessels.

Even with pre-treatment attempts to assess response, and even more so with abnormal pre-treatment evaluations of ovarian reserve, the stimulation may result in very few follicles developing, the end result may be few or no eggs obtained at egg retrieval or even cancellation of the treatment cycle prior to egg retrieval. Some research suggested that the risk of ovarian tumors may increase in women who take any fertility drugs over a long period of time. These studies had significant flaws which limited the strength of the conclusions. More recent studies have not confirmed this risk. A major risk factor for ovarian cancer is infertility per se, suggesting that early reports may have falsely attributed the risk resulting from infertility to the use of medications to overcome it. In these studies, conception lowered the risk of ovarian tumors to that of fertile women.

GnRH-agonists (Leuprolide acetate) (Lupron®): This medication is taken by injection. There are two forms of the medication: A short acting medication requiring daily injections and a long-acting preparation lasting for 1-3 months. The primary role of this medication is to prevent a premature LH surge, which could result in the release of eggs before they are ready to be retrieved. Since GnRH-agonists initially cause a release of FSH and LH from the pituitary, they can also be used to start the growth of the follicles or initiate the final stages of egg maturation. Though leuprolide acetate is an FDA (Federal Drug Administration) approved medication, it has not been approved for use in IVF, although it has routinely been used in this way for more than 20 years. Potential side effects usually experienced with long-term use include but are not limited to hot flashes, vaginal dryness, bone loss, nausea, vomiting, and skin reactions at the injection site, fluid retention, muscle aches, headaches, and depression. No long term or serious side effects are known. Since GnRH-a are oftentimes administered after ovulation, it is possible that they will be taken early in pregnancy. The safest course of action is to use a barrier method of contraception (condoms) the month you will be starting the GnRH-a. GnRH-a have not been associated with any fetal malformations however you should discontinue use of the GnRH-a as soon as pregnancy is confirmed.

GnRH-antagonists (Ganirelix Acetate or Cetrorelix Acetate) (Ganirelix®, Cetrotide®):

These are another class of medications used to prevent premature ovulation. They tend to be used for short periods of time in the late stages of ovarian stimulation. The potential side effects include, but are not limited to, abdominal pain, headaches, skin reaction at the injection site, and nausea.

Human chorionic gonadotropin (hCG) (Profasi®, Novarel®, Pregnyl®, Ovidrel®):

HCG is a natural hormone used in IVF to induce the eggs to

become mature and fertilizable. The timing of this medication is critical to retrieve mature eggs. Potential side effects include, but are not limited to breast tenderness, bloating, and pelvic discomfort.

Progesterone, and in some cases, estradiol: Progesterone and estradiol are hormones normally produced by the ovaries after ovulation. After egg retrieval in some women, the ovaries will not produce adequate amounts of these hormones for long enough to fully support a pregnancy. Accordingly, supplemental progesterone, and in some cases estradiol, are given to ensure adequate hormonal support of the uterine lining. Progesterone is usually given by injection or by the vaginal route (Endometrin®, Crinone®, Prochieve®, Prometrium®, or pharmacist-compounded suppositories) after egg retrieval. Progesterone is often continued for some weeks after a pregnancy has been confirmed. Progesterone in this natural form has not been associated with an increase in fetal abnormalities. Side effects of progesterone include depression, sleepiness, and allergic reaction and if given by intra-muscular injection includes the additional risk of infection or pain at the application site. Estradiol, if given, can be by oral, trans-dermal, intramuscular, or vaginal administration. Side effects of estradiol include nausea, irritation at the injection site if given by the trans-dermal route and the risk of blood clots or stroke.

Oral contraceptive pills: Many treatment protocols include oral contraceptive pills to be taken for 2 to 4 weeks before gonadotropin injections are started in order to suppress hormone production and bring the pituitary gland, ovaries and uterus to a basal state prior to initiating stimulation and to schedule the cycle start. Side effects include unscheduled bleeding, headache, breast tenderness, nausea, swelling and the risk of blood clots or stroke.

Other medications: Antibiotics may be given for a short time during the treatment cycle to reduce the risk of infection associated with egg retrieval or embryo transfer. Antibiotic use may be associated with causing a yeast infection, nausea, vomiting, diarrhea, rashes, sensitivity to the sun, and allergic reactions. Anti-anxiety medications or muscle relaxants may be recommended prior to the embryo transfer; the most common side effect is drowsiness. Other medications such as steroids, heparin, low molecular weight heparin or aspirin may also be included in the treatment protocol.

FERTILITY DRUGS DO NOT INCREASE RISK FOR OVARIAN CANCER

I am often asked whether the medications we use in our fertility treatments can cause ovarian cancer. In the past, conflicting stories have been published mainly in the newspapers and non medical magazines. Recently, a scientific forum, Medscape Medical News, reviewed research on this topic and the good news is summarized below.

On February 10, 2009 — It was concluded in the largest study of the subject to date that Fertility drugs do not increase the risk for ovarian cancer. There was no convincing association with ovarian cancer for any of the 4 different types of drugs used to treat infertile women — gonadotropins (Bravelle, Menopur, Gonal F, Follistim), clomiphene citrate (Clomid, Serophene), human chorionic gonadotropin (HCG, Novadrel, Ovidrel) and gonadotropin releasing hormone agonist/antagonist (Lupron, Ganirelix, Cetrotide).

Instead, the data suggest that factors related to the diagnosis of infertility (for example, genetic or biological factors) — and not the use of fertility drugs — increase the overall risk for ovarian cancer.

However, they also point out that there is a major limitation to this study — many of the participants have not yet reached the age at which the incidence of ovarian cancer peaks (early 60s).

The study, headed by Allen Jensen, PhD, assistant professor of cancer epidemiology at the Danish Cancer Society's Institute of Cancer Epidemiology, in Copenhagen, Denmark, was reported online February 5 in BMJ(British Medical Journal).

These data are reassuring but cannot absolutely rule out a very small increase in ovarian cancer or one that occurs much later in life.

Main Limitation Is Age of Participants

A link between fertility drugs and increased risk for ovarian cancer was suggested by several studies in the early 1990s, and this has created concern for patients undergoing infertility treatment. However, many of the studies over the past 8 to 10 years have been very small and none were able to reject or confirm the hypothesis.

This current study was the largest because it included 156 women with ovarian cancer, more than 3 times as many as any previous cohort.

The main limitation of the study, however, is the age of the participants. These were young women; they were first evaluated for infertility at a median age of 30 years. Despite a long follow-up, the median age of these women at the end of the follow-up period was 47 years. This is below the usual age at which women are diagnosed with ovarian cancer, which reaches a peak incidence in women in their early 60s. So there is a possibility that there could still be a spate of ovarian cancers diagnosed as these women age, which could alter the conclusions.

This is a question that nobody can answer yet, we should say that the data so far are reassuring with this observation period, and with this age of the cohort, we cannot see any association with an increase in the risk of ovarian cancer.

The researchers intend to revisit the data at regular points in the future to check on the progress of the study cohort with "passive surveillance," The Danish system of personal identification numbers and nationwide health and cancer registries will allow them to track any new diagnosis of ovarian cancer.

Cannot Exclude Small Possibility

The Danish study investigated the records of 54,362 women with infertility problems, and compared 156 women who developed invasive epithelial ovarian cancer with 1241 controls.

However, although this study was much larger than previous investigations, it still could not exclude the possibility of a small increase in the risk for ovarian cancer in users of fertility drugs, The rate ratio for use of any fertility drug was 1.03, but the upper bound of the 95% confidence interval was 1.47.

Larger numbers of women will need to be studied to answer this question, and these will come with further follow-up of the cohort as they enter the age range where ovarian cancer is most common. Some women who take fertility drugs will inevitably develop ovarian cancer by chance alone, but current evidence suggests that women who use these drugs do not have an increased risk.

Clinical Context

Infertility has previously been associated with an increased risk for ovarian cancer. In an epidemiologic study of 3837 women treated for infertility, Rossing and colleagues demonstrated that infertility increased the risk for malignant ovarian tumors by a factor of 2.5 vs. the overall community prevalence of ovarian cancer. This study, which was published in the September 22, 1994, issue of the New England Journal of Medicine, also suggested that the use of clomiphene in particular could increase the risk for ovarian cancer, particularly in women who had used the medication for more than 1 year.

The current study uses a large cohort of women to examine the effects of different fertility medications on the risk for ovarian cancer.

Study Highlights

- The study cohort consisted of women referred to Danish hospitals or infertility clinics between 1963 and 1998. A total of 54,362 women had data available for analysis.
- Cases of ovarian cancer were documented with use of 2 national registries: 176 women were diagnosed with epithelial

ovarian cancer during a median follow-up of 16 years, and 156 women had data for analysis.

- The main outcome of the study was the relationship between fertility drugs and the risk for ovarian cancer. The 156 women with ovarian cancer were compared vs. 1241 women from the infertile cohort who did not have ovarian cancer.

- The median year for entry into the infertility clinics was 1989, and the median age at the first evaluation for infertility was 30 years.

- The median time from entry into the cohort until the diagnosis of ovarian cancer was 14.5 years.

- Overall, the use of fertility drugs did not significantly affect the incidence of ovarian cancer. Fertility drugs were used by 49% and 50% of women with and without ovarian cancer, respectively.

- Clomiphene was the most widely used fertility drug, followed closely by human chorionic gonadotropins. Other gonadotropins and gonadotropin-releasing hormones were used less frequently.

- Nulliparity (No births) conferred an especially high risk for ovarian cancer in these women with infertility. The risk for ovarian cancer decreased with a higher number of births.

- The use of oral contraceptives and the cause of infertility did not significantly affect the risk for ovarian cancer.

- After adjustment for parity (Births), none of the individual fertility drugs were associated with a significant effect on the risk for ovarian cancer. The number of cycles used or the number of years since first use did not affect this conclusion.

- Similarly, combination treatment with multiple fertility drugs did not appear to increase the risk for ovarian cancer.

- Serous tumors were the most common histologic type of ovarian cancer. Clomiphene use was associated with a higher risk for serous tumor vs. no use of fertility drugs but only in women who used clomiphene at least 15 years before the diagnosis of ovarian cancer.

- Previous research has found that infertility is associated with an increased risk for ovarian cancer, particularly in women who used clomiphene for more than 12 months.
- The current study suggests that fertility drugs do not significantly increase the risk for ovarian cancer.

CO-CULTURE OF EMBRYOS OFFERED AT EAST COAST FERTILITY

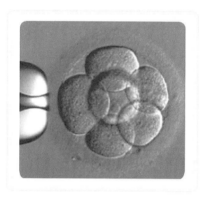

Embryo

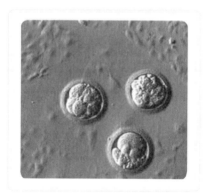

Embryos with Cumulus Cells

In the past 30 years great strides have been made in the field of in vitro fertilization (IVF). The use of ovulation induction to recruit multiple eggs increased the IVF success rate in the late 1970's. The addition of FSH and a GnRH agonist (such as Lupron) to the stimulation protocol increased success rates even more. Ultrasound-guided retrievals made the oocyte (egg) pickup less invasive, and the ultrasound-guided transfer improved the efficiency of the transfer. In the late 1990's, a culture revolution, that is in the media environment bathing and feeding the embryos, greatly improved success due to our ability to provide a healthier environment for the embryos. All these advances have had a great impact on our success rates with IVF to the point that approximately 50% of retrievals will result in a pregnancy. Unfortunately, older patients and some younger ones as well have yet to share in this success.

Many IVF programs have reintroduced the concept of utilizing a co-culture medium to improve the quality and implantation of embryos. Co-culture is a procedure whereby "helper" cells are grown along with the developing embryo. Today, the most popular cell lines include endometrial cells (from the endometrium, or uterine lining) and cumulus cells from women's ovaries. Both cell lines are derived from the patient, thereby eliminating any concerns regarding transmission of viruses. Endometrial cells are much more difficult to obtain and process, while cumulus cells are routinely removed along with the oocytes during IVF retrieval.

Cumulus cells play an important role in the maturation and development of oocytes. After ovulation cumulus cells normally produce a chemical called Hyaluronan. Hyaluronan is secreted by many cells of the body and is involved in regulating cell adhesion, growth and development. Recent evidence has shown that Hyaluronan is found normally in the uterus at the time of implantation.

Co-culture of cumulus cells provides an opportunity to detoxify the embryo's culture medium that the embryos are growing in and produce growth factors important for cell development 1,2. This may explain why some human embryos can experience improved development with the use of co-culture.

Preparation of co-culture cells starts with separation of the cumulus cells from the oocytes after aspiration of the follicles. These sheets of cells are washed thoroughly and then placed in a solution that permits the sheets to separate into individual cells. The cells are then washed again and transferred to a culture dish with medium and incubated overnight. During this time individual cells will attach to the culture dish and create junctions between adjoining cells. This communication is important for normal development. The following morning, cells are washed again and all normally fertilized oocytes (embryos) are added to the dish. Embryos are grown with the cumulus cells for a period of three days to achieve maximum benefit.

Performing co-culture of embryos has improved implantation and pregnancy rates above and beyond those seen with the IVF advances previously described. More importantly, it promises to offer advantages for those patients whose previous IVF cycles were unsuccessful.

References:

1. Barmat LI, Worrilow KC, Paynton BV. Growth factor expression by
    human oviduct and buffalo rat liver co culture cells. Fertil Steril 1997;
    67:775–9.
2. Fukui Y, McGowan LT, James RW, Pugh PA, Tervit HR. Factors
    affecting the in vitro development of blastocysts of bovine oocytes
    matured and fertilized in vitro. J Reprod Fertil 1991;92:125–31.

THINGS YOU SHOULD KNOW ABOUT YOUR EMBRYO TRANSFER

- **After a few days of development, the best appearing embryos are selected for transfer**
- **The number chosen influences the pregnancy rate and the multiple pregnancy rate**
- **A woman's age and the appearance of the developing embryo have the greatest influences on pregnancy outcome**
- **Embryos are placed in the uterine cavity with a thin tube**
- **Excess embryos of sufficient quality that are not transferred can be frozen**

After a few days of development, one or more embryos are selected for transfer to the uterine cavity. Embryos are placed in the uterine cavity with a thin tube (catheter). Ultrasound guidance may be used to help guide the catheter or confirm placement through the cervix and into the uterine cavity. Although the possibility of a complication from the embryo transfer is very rare, risks include infection and loss of, or damage to the embryos.

The number of embryos transferred influences the pregnancy rate and the multiple pregnancy rate. The age of the woman and the appearance of the developing embryo have the greatest influence on pregnancy outcome and the chance for multiple pregnancies. While it is possible by virtue of spontaneous embryo splitting, it is unusual to develop more fetuses than the number of embryos transferred. These become identical twins. It is critical to discuss with your doctor the number to be transferred before the transfer is done.

In an effort to help curtail the problem of multiple pregnancies national guidelines published in 2006 recommend limits on the number of embryos to transfer (see Tables below). These limits should be viewed as a recommendation on the number of embryos to transfer and thereby minimize the risk of a multiple pregnancy. These limits differ depending on the developmental stage of the embryos and the quality of the embryos and should take into account the patient's personal history.

Recommended limits on number of 2-3 day old embryos to transfer

Embryos	age <35	age 35-37	age 38-40	age >40
favorable	I or 2	2	3	5
unfavorable	2	3	4	5

Recommended limits on number of 5-6 day old embryos to transfer

Embryo Prognosis	age <35	age 35-37	age 38-40	age >40
favorable	I	2	2	3
unfavorable	2	2	3	3

In some cases, there will be additional embryos remaining in the lab after the transfer is completed. Depending on their pregnancy potential, it may be possible to freeze them for possible use in a subsequent cycle.

CRYOPRESERVATION OF EMBRYOS

In 1985, my mentors, Drs. Howard W. Jones Jr. and his wife Georgeanna Seegar Jones, the two pioneers of in-vitro fertilization in the USA and the entire western hemisphere, proposed the potential benefits of cryopreserving or freezing embryos following an IVF cycle. They predicted that cryopreserving embryos for future transfers would increase the overall success rate of IVF and make the procedure more efficient and cost effective. They also suggested that it would reduce the overall risks of IVF. For example, one fresh IVF cycle might yield many embryos which can be used in future frozen embryo transfer cycles, if necessary. This helps to limit the exposure to certain risks confronted only in a fresh IVF cycle such as the use of injectable stimulation hormones, the egg retrieval operation, and general anesthesia.

At East Coast Fertility, we are realizing the Jones' dream of safer, more efficient and cost effective IVF. By utilizing the ability to cryo-preserve embryos in 2007, 61.5% (118/192) of patients under 35 were successful in having a live birth as a result of only one egg stimulation and retrieval cycle! In addition, because of our outstanding Embryology Laboratory, we are usually able to transfer as few as 1 or 2 high quality embryos per cycle and avoid risky triplet pregnancies. In fact, since 2002, the only triplet pregnancies we have experienced have resulted from the successful implantation of two embryos, one of which goes on to split into identical twins (this is rare!). By cryopreserving embryos in certain high-risk circumstances, we are able to vastly reduce the risk of ovarian hyperstimulation syndrome requiring hospitalization. At East Coast Fertility, safety of our patients comes first. Fortunately, our success with frozen embryo transfers is equivalent to that of fresh embryo transfers, so that pregnancy rates are not compromised in the name of safety, nor are the babies.

Today, as reported in the Daily Science: "The results are good news as an increasing number of children, estimated to be 25% of assisted reproductive technology (ART) babies worldwide, are now born after freezing or vitrification" (a process similar to freezing that prevents the formation of ice crystals).

The study, led by Dr Ulla-Britt Wennerholm, an obstetrician at the Institute for Clinical Sciences, Sahlgrenska Academy (Goteborg, Sweden), reviewed the evidence from 21 controlled studies that reported on prenatal or child outcomes after freezing or vitrification.

She found that embryos that had been frozen shortly after they started to divide (early stage cleavage embryos) had a better, or at least as good, obstetric outcome (measured as preterm birth and low birth weight) as children born from fresh cycles of IVF (in vitro fertilization) or ICSI (intracytoplasmic sperm injection). There were comparable malformation rates between the fresh and frozen cycles. There were limited data available for freezing of blastocysts (embryos that have developed for about five days) and for vitrification of early cleavage stage embryos, blastocysts and eggs.

'Slow freezing of embryos has been used for 25 years and data concerning infant outcome seem reassuring with even higher birth weights and lower rates of preterm and low birth weights than children born after fresh IVF/ICSI. For the newly introduced technique of vitrification of blastocysts and oocytes, very limited data have been reported on obstetric and neonatal outcomes. This emphasizes the urgent need for properly controlled follow-up studies of neonatal outcomes and a careful assessment of evidence currently available before these techniques are added to daily routines. In addition, long-term follow-up studies are needed for all cryopreservation techniques,' concluded Dr Wennerholm.

The use of frozen embryos has become a common standard of care in most IVF Programs. At East Coast Fertility we are able to keep multiple pregnancy rates down - by only transferring one or two embryos at a time - while allowing patients to hold on to the additional embryos that they may have created during the fresh cycle. It is like creating an insurance plan for patients. We developed a unique financial incentive program using the technology of cryo-preservation to encourage patients to transfer only one healthy embryo at a time. In order to ensure the best out come for mother and child - these special pricing plans take the burden off the patient to pay for the additional transfers and the cryo- preservation process. We have eliminated the cost of cryopreservation, storage and embryo transfer for patients in the single embryo transfer program. Thus, patients no longer have that financial pressure to put all their eggs in one basket! We truly believe we are practicing the most successful, safe and cost effective IVF utilizing cryopreservation.

WAYS TO DEAL WITH STRESS AND OPTIMIZE PREGNANCY SUCCESS

NOMINATED FOR BEST SUPPORTING ROLE IS…

MANY husbands complain that they feel left out of the whole IVF process as all the attention and care is apparently directed towards the woman. If anything they may feel that at best they can show up for the retrieval at which time they are expected to donate their sperm on demand. If you should fail at this then all the money, time, hope and efforts were wasted all because you choked when you could not even perform this one "simple" step. I have not witnessed the terror and horrors of war but I have seen the devastation resulting from an IVF cycle failed as a result of a husband's inability to collect a specimen. Relationships often do not survive in the wake of such a disappointment. Talk about performing under pressure, there is more at stake in the collection room than pitching in the World Series. Husbands view IVF from a different perspective than their wives. They are not the ones being injected with hormones; commuting to the physician's office frequently over a two week span for blood tests and vaginal ultrasounds and undergoing a transvaginal needle aspiration. At least women are involved in the entire process, speak with and see the IVF staff regularly and understand what they are doing and are deeply invested emotionally and physically in this experience. So what is a husband to do?

Get Involved

Those couples that appear to deal best with the stress of IVF are ones that do it together. Many husbands learn to give their wives the injections. It helps involve them in the efforts and give them some degree of control over the process. They can relate better to what their wives are doing and take pride that they are contributing towards the common goal of achieving the baby. When possible, husbands should accompany their wives to the doctor visits. They can interact with the staff, get questions answered and obtain a better understanding of what is going on. This not only makes women feel like their husbands are supportive but is helpful in getting accurate information and directions. Both of these things are so important that in a husband's absence I would recommend a surrogate such as a friend, sister, or mother to be there if he cannot be. Support from him and others help diminish the level of stress and especially if it comes from the husband helps to solidify their relationship.

Husbands should accompany their wives to the embryo transfer. This can be a highly emotional procedure. Your embryo/s is being placed in the womb and at least in that moment many women feel as if they are pregnant. Life may be starting here and it is wonderful for a husband to share this moment with his wife. Perhaps he may keep the Petri dish as a keepsake as the "baby's first crib". It is an experience a couple is not likely to forget as their first time together as a family.

With regards to the pressure of performing to provide the specimen at the time of the retrieval, I would recommend that a husband freeze a specimen collected on a previous day when he does not have the intense pressure of having to produce at that moment or else. Having the insurance of a back up frozen specimen takes much of the pressure off at the time of retrieval making it that much easier to produce a fresh specimen. There are strategies that can be planned for special circumstances including arranging for assistance from your wife and using collection condoms so that the specimen can be collected during intercourse. Depending on the program these alternatives may be available.

I LOOK PRETTY
GOOD IN SCRUBS

The experience husbands feel when going through an IVF cycle varies depending in large part on how involved they get. Not only will it help relieve much of the stress for your wife and your relationship the more involved you are but you will feel more invested in it and more in control over the outcome. Many husbands pride themselves in their new found skill with mixing hormonal medications and administering injections for their wives. It helps many men who are used to caring for their wife to be in control of administering the medication for them. Successful IVF becomes something they play a very active role in and relate better to the experience, their wife and the resulting baby. Despite your lack of prior experience, most people can learn to prepare and administer the medication. Whether it is the feeling of "playing doctor" or the knowledge that you are contributing significantly in the process and supporting your wife, most men relate to me that giving their wives the injections was a positive experience for them and for their relationship.

Along the same line of thinking, accompanying your wife at the time of embryo transfer can be most rewarding. This can be a highly emotional procedure. Your embryo/s is being placed in the womb and at least in that moment many women feel as if they are pregnant. Life may be starting here and it is wonderful to share this moment with your wife. Perhaps you may keep the Petri dish as a keepsake as the "baby's first crib". It is an experience the two of you are not likely to forget as your first time together as a family. I strongly recommend that you don those scrubs, hat and booties and join your wife as the physician transfers the embryos from the dish into her womb. Nine months later do the same at delivery for memories that last a lifetime.

IS THIS STRESS MAKING ME LOOK FAT?

I'm racing a 40 foot sailboat in 25 to 30 NNW winds yesterday out of Manhasset Bay. Gear was breaking, sails ripping, we broached twice....nearly did a "death roll" (when the boat gets knocked down and the tip of the mast nearly hits the water). A competitor had a man overboard; the USCG and NCPD were involved with another boat in distress. It was insane. The adrenaline is pumping, the testosterone is flowing and I walk in the door 12 hours after I left and there is Gina. She is sitting on the couch watching reruns of 90210. I just spent 10 hours engaged in manly man activity in conditions that no one intentionally goes out in and I am hyped to share it with my wife. But nooooo she is on the edge of her seat fully engrossed in a show that went off the air 12 freaking years ago....she knows what happens. Her man just returns from the sea and she cant be bothered, I lose it....I get nuts....she yells back and then without notice gets all weepy. Suddenly, as quickly as the tears came, they are gone and she is glaring at me with a look that bores right through me and in a voice similar to Linda Blair's (just as her head does a 360 in The Exorcist) says, "I took 15 *&% &^%$ pills today and 12 of them went in my @#&! Vagina, where they still are and I feel like a G*D damn gumball machine....let me put just one in your *@#(* Penis. Man I spun on my heels thinking, "why that couldn't have been me who went overboard?"

This is one husband's story about living with a woman on hormones.

It is not always this dramatic but the stress can be very difficult for a couple and many relationships benefit from professional support when going through fertility treatments. Imagine dealing with the stress, frustrations and cyclic disappointment couples feel when trying unsuccessfully to start a family. Add to this that your wife is being pumped up with hormones that have the potential to lower her threshold of rationality and sanity. Outbursts of anger directed at especially those closest to them are very common. Under normal circumstances most of us can control our reactions without letting our emotions get in the way. Hormones can greatly diminish our ability to control our behavior when circumstances become tense and stressful. Hormones have even been used as a defense in murder cases. My recommendation is to get rid of any guns in the house and not respond to apparent emotional outbursts. This should pass when the cycle is completed and the hormones have faded from the system. If not...?

TIPS FOR REDUCING INFERTILITY STRESS

These are tips I recently read on a post by Melissa Brisman (source: theadventurouswriter.com) for reducing infertility stress and will help if you're trying to get pregnant and are coping with constant disappointment! You're probably getting a little stressed out - and that definitely won't help you conceive. These stress relief tips may increase your chances of getting pregnant, and will definitely improve your mood and relationships.

Before the tips, here's a hopeful quip:

"Slow down and everything you are chasing will come around and catch you," said John De Paola.

I don't know if pregnancy will "catch" you if you slow down… but heck, it's worth a try! To learn more about sperm, ovulation, and getting pregnant, click Fertility and Infertility for Dummies by Gillian Lockwood and others. And, read on for dozens of tips on reducing the stress of infertility….At East Coast Fertility, join our Mind Body Program where reducing stress and improving your odds is the name of the game.

Social Ways to Reduce Infertility Stress

- Tell your friends what you need. If don't want people to keep asking if you're pregnant (I hate that!), then tell them that you'll give them the good news when you're ready!

- Accept your way of dealing with infertility. You and your partner's method of coping with infertility could be much different than mine, or your sister's - and the sooner that you accept it, the better.
- Talk to your friends about your frustrations and joys.
- Have a relaxing glass of wine or a margarita with friends, but don't overdo it (though some say you shouldn't drink alcohol at all when you're trying to get pregnant...that's a personal choice).
- Prioritize invitations to reduce stress. Give yourself time to unwind and do what you want to do. Say no to parties or get-togethers, or just make a brief appearance.
- Don't fall into the trap of comparing your life, situation, relationship, or family to other people's.

Physical Ways to Reduce Infertility Stress

- Get a full-body massage - and tell your massage therapist that you're trying to get pregnant.
- Spend time out in nature: walking, skating skiing in the winter, hiking in the summer.
- Take a warm bubble bath (but if you're a female or male coping with infertility, make sure you check with your doctor first).
- Stop eating before you're full - don't gorge on chocolates, chips, or fast food.
- Get enough sleep.
- Reduce your caffeine intake (I'm sure you've heard that before!).
- Take your vitamins, supplements, minerals (you've heard that before, too, I bet).
- Drinks lots of water.
- Get a manicure or pedicure.
- Make love for the sake of making love.

Mental Ways to Reduce Infertility Stress

- Volunteer at a food bank, hospital, or animal shelter.
- Take downtime to snooze, read, and relax.
- Play your favorite card and board games - laughing will reduce the stress of getting pregnant.
- Take a regular crossword puzzle or Sudoku break.
- Pick your battles, choose your priorities.
- Let go of the little stuff.
- Watch your favorite TV shows or movies.
- Share your baking or meals with homebound people or lonely neighbors.

Emotional Ways to Reduce Infertility Stress

- Practice gratitude.
- Have realistic expectations.
- Laugh!
- Stay in touch with your authentic emotions.
- Cry, scream, or punch the pillow when you need to.
- Stop to take a deep breath every hour or so throughout the day.
- Let yourself grieve. Reducing stress involves expressing your emotions.
- Keep your old traditions and healthy habits alive, but be open to new ones.

Creative Ways to Reduce Infertility Stress

- Paint, draw or carve your thoughts and feelings.
- Visit a museum or art gallery to reduce holiday stress.
- Go to a movie in the middle of the day by yourself.
- Listen to music that relaxes and/or energizes you.
- Go for a drive in the country; stop for hot chocolate and muffins.
- Write in your journal to reduce stress.

Spiritual Ways to Reduce Infertility Stress

- Pray, and remember the big picture.
- Read the Bible, Torah, or other meaningful book.
- Seek the deep meaning behind church or mass services to reduce holiday stress.
- Remember that your God, Creator or Higher Power is working behind the scenes.
- Adjust your perspective to include peace, compassion, and forgiveness.

Family Ways to Reduce Infertility Stress

- Change your regular responses to aggravating family members, especially if your normal responses haven't worked in the past!
- Shrug off challenges and criticisms.
- Let go of past betrayals, mistakes, failures - both yours and others'.
- Don't expect people to change (unless you change first).
- Maintain healthy boundaries to reduce infertility stress.

Readers, how do you let go of the stress of trying to get pregnant? I find that walking in the woods out behind our house is hugely relaxing - it reminds me that life can be beautiful even without kids. There's something about deep breaths of fresh air that energize me, no matter how bad I'm feeling...

FERTILITY AND THE MIND & BODY CONNECTION

by: Bina Benisch, M.S., R.N.

At East Coast Fertility, we understand the emotional aspect that accompanies infertility, and we believe it is equally important to support our patients emotionally as well as physically. It is important to understand fertility holistically. In addition to treating the various physical etiologies of infertility, we must take into account the effects of stress and anxiety. Your mind and body work together, not separately. Therefore your thoughts have a direct effect on your physiology. When you are experiencing stress, your brain releases stress hormones. These stress hormones function in many ways. One of the stress hormones, cortisol, has been documented to interfere with the release of the reproductive hormones, GnRH (gonadotropin releasing hormone), LH (luteinizing hormone), FSH (follicle stimulating hormone), estrogen, and progesterone. In fact, severe enough stress can completely inhibit the reproductive system. Cortisol levels have also been linked to very early pregnancy loss. For this reason, it has been found extremely helpful when treating infertility, to include mind/body methods and strategies which help to alleviate the stress response that sets off a cascade of hormonal responses which may inhibit fertility.

The mind/body work we teach here at East Coast Fertility includes methods that allow the body to return to a calm and relaxed state, thereby turning off the biochemical stress response and allowing our hormonal physiology to function optimally. Feelings of anxiety, depression, isolation, and anger are common themes in infertility. Often, anger masks the feelings of loss experienced month after month of trying to conceive without success. Infertility impacts on one's marriage, self-esteem, sexual relationship, family, friends, job, and financial security.

One study showed that women going through infertility experience as much depression as women who have been diagnosed with life-threatening illnesses such as metastatic cancer, heart disease, or HIV. When women face these other illnesses, they are likely to seek out the support of their friends and family. The sad aspect of infertility is that although these women are as depressed as those facing life-threatening illnesses, they are far less likely to seek out support from friends and family. Often, thoughts of not living up to the expectation to become pregnant, thoughts such as "why is this happening to me?!", and the intense emotions of loss related to the thought that one may never have a child, lead to feelings of isolation, anger, and depression.

Although there is a correlation between stress and infertility, the relationship remains complex. However, the research does in fact suggest that psychosocial factors such as depression and anxiety correlate with lower pregnancy rates following IVF. In addition, of the women who participated in Alice Domar's Mind/Body program at the Mind/Body institute in Boston, 55% conceived pregnancies that resulted in the birth of a full term baby compared with 20% of the control group.

~ Mind/Body Support Group at East Coast Fertility ~

In our Mind/Body support group, patients experience the opportunity to share information, feelings, or their own personal stories. You may be surprised to see how your support can help others or you may be relieved to hear others experiencing the same type of thoughts and feelings as you experience. Often, the supportive nature of this group, and the connection that develops between members, fosters a healing process. Feelings of isolation, anger, and stress are slowly relieved.

Our Mind/Body program focuses on symptom reduction and

developing a sense of control over one's life by utilizing Mind/Body strategies and interventions which elicit the relaxation response. The relaxation response is actually a physical state that counteracts the stress response. You can think of it as the physiological opposite of the body's stress response. We cannot be stressed and relaxed at the same time. Therefore when a person elicits the relaxation response, the body's stress response is halted, stress hormones diminish. Stress responses such as heart rate, metabolic rate, blood pressure, and shallow breathing decrease. Breathing becomes slower and deeper, so we have more oxygen being delivered to all the cells in the body. The way in which you are taught to elicit the relaxation response is through methods such as: breath focus, guided visual imagery, muscle Relaxation and learned mindfulness, and meditation.

In Mind/Body work, we also work with "cognitive restructuring" which is examining our negative thoughts, seeing where there is distortion, and reframing our thoughts positively and realistically. Often, we have held on to certain negative thoughts and feelings we may have developed years ago. The thought pattern becomes so ingrained in us, that we take it for truth, when in fact, it is a distortion. Cognitive restructuring will help you examine your thoughts and see which are distorted, causing you needless worry, anxiety, or depression. Once you understand how a thought is distorted, you can change those thoughts and alleviate the anxiety attached to them.

Awareness of the mind/body connection allows us to use our minds to make changes in our physiology. This holistic treatment - combining bio-medical science with mind/body medicine deals with the treatment of the whole individual rather than looking only at the physical aspect. The fact is body and mind work together. We invite you to take advantage of this unique area of support provided at East Coast Fertility and join our Mind/Body group.

ALTERNATIVE THERAPIES AND HOLISTIC MEDICINE

Stress induces a "fight or flight" response in the body. Our thoughts stimulate various centers in the brain connected to organs in our body. The sympathetic nervous system is activated; increasing our heart rate, respirations, etc. The endocrine system simultaneously releases hormones into the blood stream. The adrenal gland is stimulated and adrenaline is released. For example, when you are having a nightmare, your brain believes that this is real when it in fact is not. Nevertheless, our bodies still react to the threat as if it is real with the "fight or flight" stress response.

When patients are exposed to prolonged stress, they become exhausted, they develop decreased resistance and a person's organ systems may not function optimally. Pregnancy rates may be handicapped by this condition resulting from prolonged stress. What can we do to overcome the problems resulting from the stress?

First, just breathe, meditate and calm yourself down. There are strategies available to help you and your wife deal with stress. Complimentary or alternative therapies such as meditation, massage, yoga, acupuncture and even chiropractic can help patients to relax. Psychological support groups are another way to help individuals and couples relax when facing the stress of infertility and fertility treatments. Acupuncture and chiropractic care are alternative services that are designed to help the body heal itself. The use of acupuncture for infertility dates back over 2000

years with Chinese medicine. The wisdom accumulated over genera-
tions of experience of using acupuncture has been shown to improve
fertility rates in some studies and unlock a woman's potential for health
and healing. It appears to increase the blood flow to the uterus and
perhaps relax it thereby improving the chances that an embryo may
implant into the uterine wall. In Chinese medicine, Qi is a life force
that increases with acupuncture improving an individual's balance that
improves functionality and helps conception. In western medicine we
refer to the reduction in stress and anxiety reducing the "fight or flight"
response improving the function of a woman's organ systems.

Chiropractic care focuses on the function of the nervous system
which controls all the functions of the body. An interference with the
nervous system will result in a dysfunction to an area of the body and
decrease health. Every level of the spine can be related to a fertility function. Subluxations or malalignments of the spine can abnormally impact
the nerves leading to the reproductive organs and pituitary gland. State
of the art electromyography and thermal scans can diagnose when the
nervous system is disturbed. A diagnostic scan can be a valuable tool in
helping a physician to understand some fertility problems not typically
noted in routine workups. The use of chiropractic has the potential to
improve fertility handicapped by suboptimal alignment of the spine.

We have seen great success with our Mind-Body Support program.
An improvement in pregnancy rates has been demonstrated in a study
presented at the American Society of Reproductive Medicine. Strategies
are taught to help reduce the effects of stress while going through an
IVF cycle. Support groups allow patients to meet persons going through
similar experiences and with whom they may share their stories and
burdens.

Prayer can also be helpful. A patient recommended contemplation
of the following to others experiencing the stress of IVF. "God grant me
the serenity to accept the things I cannot change, the courage to change
the things I can, and the wisdom to know the difference".

CONTEMPORARY ISSUES IN INFERTILITY

A DOZEN EMBRYOS, WHO WILL STOP THIS MADNESS?

JUST when I thought it was safe to go back to my office at East Coast Fertility, a little over 5 months post Octomom, I was confronted once again with shocking news. This time it was a record breaking 12 embryos implanted. Eight is alarming and wrong, a dozen just five months later makes me wonder how such a horrific result could be possible. Who let this happen?

Octomom was a result of IVF with an embryo transfer of six embryos. This far exceeds the number that the Society of Assisted Reproductive Technology (SART) has recommended as the limit. Physicians have known for many years the dangers of multiple pregnancies and have worked steadily to formulate evidence—based guidelines for the number of embryos to transfer in IVF cycles. The current rate of triplets in IVF cycles nationally has dropped in 2005 to only 2% of cycles. At East Coast Fertility our triplet rate has been below 1% since 2002 and not one of these occurred from transfer of more than 2 embryos.

However, the Tunisian woman who is expecting six male and six female babies conceived using gonadotropins in combination with insemination. Unfortunately, one does not have the same control with insemination as you do with IVF. As many eggs as is stimulated by the gonadotropin injections can implant with intrauterine insemination (IUI) or without the benefit of retrieval of the eggs as one performs as part of the IVF procedure. With IVF one can limit the number of embryos transferred to a woman's uterus. Insurance companies do not typically cover IVF but are more likely to cover IUIs. However, if one considers the cost of multiple pregnancy; including hospitalization for mother and babies born prematurely requiring the neonatal intensive care unit (NICU) and care for babies born handicapped, it would be a lot cheaper for insurance companies and employers, the government and society to cover IVF and have the control to prevent these high risk multiple pregnancies.

The dozen babies happened because the safer alternative, IVF was not performed. Gonadotropins without IVF are dangerously risky due to this lack of control over how many eggs may fertilize and implant. By virtue of insurance coverage for IUI but not for IVF, patients are encouraged to undergo gonadotropin therapy without the protection of IVF. If IVF was covered by a patient's health insurance, physicians would not need to administer gonadotropins in such a dangerous and risky way. Perhaps gonadotropin treatment without IVF should be limited to situations where the risk is minimal such as with older women who have diminished ovarian reserve. Again, if IVF is a covered alternative, who would not choose the safer, more successful treatment?

That brings us to regulating how many embryos to transfer as Octomom went through IVF with transfer of six embryos. At East Coat Fertility, a financial incentive is offered to patients to transfer a single embryo. Cryopreservation of embryos is offered for free as well as storage for patients in the Single Embryo Transfer Program. In addition, patients may return for their frozen embryo transfers for free until a baby is born. Patients are encouraged by this program not to put all their eggs in one basket. Success rates with a fresh single embryo transfer with IVF at our program, is nearly 50%.

If IVF were a covered service as I recommend thereby avoiding the dangers of uncontrolled gonadotropin use without IVF then we need to regulate how many embryos are transferred. The SART recommendations regarding the number to transfer should be made law to prevent such aberrations as Octomom from happening. There is flexibility built into the recommendations taking into account critical factors such as patient age and embryo quality. One can even factor in past experience. I believe it is not until we discourage the use of gonadotropins without IVF by offering IVF as a regulated covered alternative will we eliminate risky multiple pregnancies. Until then, all of us including society, the government, insurance companies and employers are to blame for letting these dangerous multiple pregnancies occur.

NO MORE "JON AND KATE" CASUALTIES

The Jon and Kate Plus Eight story has brought the tragedy of the high order multiple pregnancy to the American living room. This is a subject that I was first introduced to when I entered the field of reproductive endocrinology and infertility in 1985 at the Jones Institute in Virginia. In those days, fertility treatments, like IVF were inefficient and we needed to transfer multiple embryos to ensure a reasonable chance for successful implantation. In 1985 a favorite patient of mine conceived with quadruplets. I lived through the pregnancy related issues she experienced, the birth and subsequent difficulties with some of the babies. There were numerous operations, hospitalizations and this added tremendous stress in their lives and in their marriage.

Over the years, I have seen many high order multiple pregnancies, a side effect of transferring excessive numbers of embryos with an inefficient procedure. I have experienced through my patients, pregnancy complications, antenatal and postnatal demise and difficulties and complications suffered by the babies. Many of these marriages failed to survive the stresses, some of the patients suffered depression and there were many issues with the babies.

I still feel the pains I experienced with my patients during those early years of IVF. We infertility doctors were responsible for many high order multiple pregnancies that often did not end well. And I carry that in my heart. When I opened East Cost Fertility, I swore that I would not be responsible again for any conception greater than twins. The only triplets I have had since 2002 are from an embryo transfer of two where the embryos split and created a third baby. I don't ever want to be responsible for anything like that again. Then IVF was inefficient, today, the implantation rates are far superior. There is no excuse for octomom or sextuplets like Kate has had. I don't feel gonadotropins with IUI are as safe as IVF where you can limit the number of embryos. We need to enforce the guidelines provided by the American Society of Reproductive Medicine so that programs and patients are compelled to be responsible and limit risk. There is a competitive pressure felt by IVF programs to transfer more embryos as their statistics and success rates are inspected by prospective patients. Programs have not uniformly followed these guidelines. It is only through outside regulation that we can prevent the cause of these high order multiple pregnancies.

I started the Single Embryo Transfer program at East Coast Fertility to encourage patients to limit the number of embryos replaced into the uterus to one in good prognosis patients by eliminating the financial factor. These patients are offered free cryopreservation, embryo storage and frozen embryo transfers so there is no financial pressure for patients to put all their eggs in one basket. This represents a savings of up to over $12,000 and ensures a better chance of a healthy pregnancy and healthy baby. It is my sincere hope that situations that led to the sextuplets of Jon and Kate and octomom are eliminated through regulations and financial incentives such as the Single Embryo Transfer program.

WHY "THE WYDEN BILL" DOES NOT SUPPORT INFERTILITY PATIENTS

Patients often seek my help, desperate to try In-Vitro Fertilization (IVF) after having a previous cycle cancelled at an outside clinic. These patients stimulated with fewer follicles and therefore due to their lower pregnancy expectations were not allowed to proceed. We presented our data on IVF performed on patients with 3 or fewer follicles at the American Society for Reproductive Medicine (ASRM) in 2008. Our pregnancy rate was 15% for this group. Though this is admittedly low, for those who were successful in having a baby using their own eggs it was felt by them to be miraculous because they were either not allowed to cycle at other centers or had their cycles cancelled.

We counseled them regarding their lower odds for success but some elected to give it a try. Previously, most of these patients were offered Intra-Uterine Insemination (IUI), a much less successful option that does not affect the programs reportable pregnancy rates.

Unlike most other fields in medicine, IVF results are subject to public reporting since the passage of the Wyden Bill in 1992. http://www1.wfubmc.edu/NR/rdonlyres/42443A72-266B-466A-B08F-363230558FE1/0/pspring98.pdf). The intent of the CDC (Center for Disease Control) report and SART (Society of Reproductive

Technology) report was to help infertility patients by informing them of the relative success of different IVF programs. Unfortunately, what sometimes creates the best IVF statistical outcomes in pregnancy rates is not always what is in the best interest of the mother, child, family and society (http://www.thefertilityadvocate.com/wpblog/?p=1573). Now that prospective patients are comparing pregnancy rates between programs there is a competitive pressure on these programs to produce the best reportable rates. This means that patients with lower odds of success are less likely to be offered IVF retrievals and are diverted to IUIs or donor egg cycles.

The high order multiple birth rate was also fueled by competition in the field to have the highest success rates. The Wyden Bill results in competitive pressure to transfer more embryos to increase the pregnancy rate as reported. Despite the fact that there is evidence that a program can achieve similar live birth rates by transferring a single embryo each time, the Wyden Bill creates a disincentive to do so. It is no surprise that the clinics with the highest success rates have also had the highest triplet rates. Live birth rates are reported per fresh cycle and those from subsequent frozen embryo transfers are not included. It is true that live birth rates are reported for frozen embryo transfers separately but again it is per transfer motivating programs to transfer multiple embryos to enhance their success rates. If live birth rates were reported per fresh IVF stimulation and retrieval (that part of IVF with risk) including those conceived from subsequent frozen embryo transfers then programs would be likely to provide the less risky option of single embryo transfer to patients.

William Petok, Ph.D the Chair of The American Fertility Association's Education Committee reported on Single Embryo Transfer (SET) "Single Embryo Transfer: Why Not Put All of Your Eggs in One Basket?". He stated that "at the ASRM meeting in November of 2008 … data was reported that looks favorably at SET. A Center for Disease Control researcher said that although multiple rather than single embryo transfer for in-vitro fertilization is less expensive in the short run, the risk of costly complications is much greater. Universal adoption of single embryo transfer would cost patients an extra $100 million to achieve the same pregnancy rates as multiple embryo transfer, but this approach would save a total of $1 billion in healthcare costs."

The risks of prematurity and pregnancy complications are far higher in multiple pregnancies than in singleton pregnancies. The financial and emotional costs to families and society are enormous. These multiple pregnancies result in much longer hospitalizations, NICU admissions, complications resulting in handicapped children and occasionally death. They often do not have a happy end including increasing the incidence of divorce. So does it not behoove insurance companies to make IVF available in such a way that encourages SET? Should not the government enforce the recommendations of SART regarding the number of embryos to transfer?

At ECF, we have, since 2006 offered our Single Embryo Transfer program to cover the financial cost for transferring one embryo at a time. For the fee of one IVF cycle, we offer free cryopreservation, embryo storage and unlimited frozen embryo transfers until a patient achieves a live birth.

We offer MicroIVF, minimal stimulation IVF, for $3900, less than the cost of 2 IUIs with three times the success rate and ¼ the risk of hyper stimulation syndrome. Since minimal stimulation does not result in as many eggs, many programs are uncomfortable offering it and therefore lowering their reported pregnancy rates.

If we are going to report pregnancy rates with IVF as is required by the Wyden Bill, let us put all programs on the same playing field by enforcing the number of embryos to be transferred and promoting minimal stimulation IVF as a safer and more efficient treatment than IUI.

The Wyden Bill without the teeth to regulate such things as the number of embryos transferred and reporting success per stimulation and retrieval and not by isolated embryo transfer does more harm than good. Let us support efforts to reduce the number of embryos transferred by removing the added costs to the patient of cryo-preservation, storage and subsequent frozen embryo transfers and by absorbing them ourselves as a profession. This will go a long way in eliminating multiple birth pregnancies, and will do the right thing for the patients, their families and for society. It's time for us doctors to "Man Up".

GIFT OF LIFE AND ITS PRICE

IVF has been responsible for 1 million babies born worldwide who otherwise without the benefit of IVF may never have been. This gift of life comes with a steep price tag that according to the NY Times article, "Gift of Life and Its Price" Sunday, October 11, 2009, hits $1 Billion per year for premature IVF babies. This price tag does not include the emotional hardships, developmental problems and permanent handicaps resulting from these premature deliveries almost always caused by multiple embryo transfer induced multiple pregnancies.

According to the Center for Disease Control, reported in the same NY Times issue, thousands of premature deliveries would be prevented resulting in a $1.1 Billion savings if elective single embryo transfer was performed on good prognosis patients. That brings us to regulating how many embryos to transfer as Octomom went through IVF with transfer of six embryos. At East Coat Fertility, we make it cost neutral to transfer only one embryo at a time by offering free cryopreservation, free embryo storage and free embryo transfers until a patient achieves a live birth, all for the cost of a single IVF cycle. Patients are encouraged by this program not to put all their eggs in one basket. Success rates with an elective fresh single embryo transfer with IVF at our program, is 50% and with subsequent frozen embryo transfers it is over 64%. It is possible that East Coast Fertility is the only center in the country doing this. That is the shame of it.

Fertility treatment without IVF is even more hazardous since as many eggs that are developed with treatment may implant and lead to a hazardous multiple pregnancy. In a perfect world, where a patient's welfare was put before insurance companies, IVF would be a covered service for all people, and the use of fertility medications in an uncontrolled IUI cycle would not be used anymore. In this perfect world, we would also regulate how many embryos are transferred. It is time to put our professional recommendations of the Society of Assisted Reproductive Technology (SART) into law. There is flexibility built into the recommendations taking into account critical factors such as patient age, embryo quality and past experience.

It is not until we discourage the use of gonadotropins without IVF by offering IVF as a regulated covered alternative will we eliminate risky multiple pregnancies. Until then, all of us including society, the government, insurance companies and employers are to blame for letting these dangerous multiple pregnancies occur.

WHEN ARE YOU TOO OLD TO BE A MOTHER?

When I saw that Maria de Carmen Bousada (the oldest mother to conceive with donated eggs and the help of an IVF program) had died, my first thought was to extend my sincere condolences to her family and in particular to her two year twin boys. My heart truly went out to them. It is a great tragedy when a death occurs especially when it is the mother of such young children. I hope and pray that Maria's family and friends find the strength to replace the love and nurturing typically given by a mother to her child. My second thought as a fertility doctor was that once again – the world of infertility was making the news because we continue to push the edges of what society views as acceptable.

This is one of the hardest things about being a doctor in a cutting edge field such as reproductive medicine. We are often put in the position of making decisions with our patients that have even bigger implications to society than the individual patient. I do my best to look at each patient, and each situation individually, but I do rely on my patients to treat me as honestly as I treat them. It is a two way street – and unfortunately, Maria lied to the clinic about her age, telling them she was only 53 years of age.

Questions are being raised regarding the responsibility of the IVF program to verify the veracity of information supplied to them by their patients in addition to confirming their health condition to carry a pregnancy.

Others add that beyond a certain age, it is unnatural to become a mother and it puts the family at risk that she may not be around to help raise the child as what occurred in this case, or even if she is perhaps she lacks the energy and stamina to raise the child properly.

At East Coast Fertility, we have a cutoff of age 50 which is admittedly random and that limit is often broken when faced with an energetic couple with a woman who passes her stress test, medical and high risk maternal fetal medicine clearances. We recently celebrated our latest 54 year old patient's delivery of a healthy baby that was highly reported in the press.

As I said, it is a struggle to separate my own personal feelings about the proper age to have a child which may be inappropriate for others who have a completely different perspective. My responsibility as the physician offering assistance to patients in need of help with procreation is to the health of my patients, the well being of the child and for the good of society.

Many women in their 50's have the health and energy to carry a pregnancy and bear a child with no more increased risk than many woman 10-20 years younger whose interest in achieving pregnancy we would never consider questioning. That being said what about the risk that the mother may not still be around to raise the child to maturity. There is no question that a young healthy couple with sufficient financial support and emotional maturity is ideal for raising a family. But, happy, successful families can take on many different faces. Single parent families exist, survive and often thrive. One can never be certain that the condition of the couple at the time of conception will continue through the child's birth or for that matter until the child has reached maturity. We do not know that a healthy woman of 30, 40 or 50 may not develop a lethal disease before a child has grown up. In addition, at least 50% of couples in the United States become divorced. One can argue that couples at risk of divorce should not get pregnant. I do not think that society is ready to conclude that any of these women should not be allowed to procreate.

So, what about the clinic's responsibility regarding confirming that a patient is giving them truthful information? We have been deceived in the past that a couple who is requesting fertility assistance was unmarried when in fact at least one partner was married to someone else. This issue is especially acute as it can raise potential liability to the clinic. As in the case of Maria de Carmen Bousada, she lied about her age and perhaps was beyond the limit the doctors and society was comfortable assisting.

For me and for our program we have raised our bar to do the proper due diligence realizing that we will not be able to get the truth in all cases but minimize the risk that we missed picking up a crucial lie. But I don't want to be "The Fertility Police". I am a fertility doctor – and my job is to help people have families no matter how different those families may look to you and me.

OCTOMOM

The American public has been stunned by the news of a mother of six giving birth to octuplets. This shocking news is compounded by the stories broadcast by the mass media regarding the woman's family situation and that she used IVF for these pregnancies.

Physicians have known for many years the dangers of multiple pregnancies and have worked steadily to formulate evidence—based guidelines for the number of embryos to transfer in IVF cycles. The current rate of triplets in IVF cycles nationally has dropped in 2005 to only 2% of cycles. At East Coast Fertility our triplet rate has been below 1% since 2002 and not one of these occurred from transfer of more than 2 embryos. In fact a financial incentive is offered to patients to transfer a single embryo. Cryopreservation of embryos is offered for free as well as storage. In addition, frozen embryo transfers are offered for free until a baby is born. Patients are encouraged by this program not to put all their eggs in one basket. Unfortunately, this was not the case for this woman. Success rates with IVF, especially, in the good prognosis patients exceed 50% even when 1 or 2 embryos are transferred. It is hard to imagine a situation where it would make sense to take such an extraordinary risk like was done in this case in California.

We should keep this case in mind when considering how many embryos to transfer. It is rarely worth the risk to put more embryos back when one can alternatively keep the embryos in frozen storage until a patient is ready to conceive again.

FERTILITY DOCTOR DENOUNCED FOR CLAIMS OF HUMAN CLONING

Source: www.ivf.net

First Octomom and now this; how shocking can the news get? I get the impression there are fertility specialists out to ruin the reputation of IVF for the rest of us. In the case of octomom, there is some question as to how the patient was counseled. At East Coast Fertility, we focus on high success with the least risk as possible. It is unfortunate that a few others aspire to something other than their patient's best interests. It is very difficult for a fertility specialist to deal with patients who insist on using up all their embryos in one attempt. We share with the patient a desire not to discard embryos but retain responsibility for not allowing potentially dangerous outcomes.

Cloning is an ethical dilemma yet to be solved by society. Until then we do not participate in cloning since we are unsure whether to do so is ethically sound. Benefits of modified forms of cloning have been proposed. Multiplying high quality embryos in patients would theoretically increase their success rates. Women who had poor quality eggs (cytoplasm) could have their nuclei transplanted into the egg of a healthy young woman. Again, theoretically, this can improve success rates.

Another proposed clinical use is to produce tissue for transplantation say in a child with cancer who requires chemotherapy.

The form of cloning that usually comes to mind however, is the creation of an identical being whether it be to replace a loved lost child or in our common vernacular a "mini me". It is this possible use of the technology that causes almost universal disdain in our society. We have yet to figure out whether there is a place for any of the aforementioned forms of cloning that is potentially more palatable.

IVF is a clinically useful form of technology that is allowing for greater than 40,000 more babies to be born each year who may otherwise never have been given life. But, as with all technology there are risks and potential downsides that need to be considered. Today, cloning as well as high ordered multiple embryo transfers moves the IVF technology beyond our comfort zone with our assessment of the potential risks and downsides. Let us not distort the relative benefit vs. risk of IVF technology by wrongfully applying it to cloning or high order multiple embryo transfer.

FERTILITY TREATMENT DURING THIS ECONOMIC DOWNTURN

Financial hardships have increased fertility challenges for many couples attempting to build their families. According to a new study release at the ASRM meeting in Atlanta last week, the recession has severely affected access to fertility treatment in this country.

Fifty eight percent of infertile couples who chose not to pursue therapy cited cost as the primary reason. About 7 percent of couples with frozen embryos discarded them from October 2008 to March 2009, representing a nearly three time increase from the prior six months. Fifty seven percent of egg donors in 2008 planned to use the money they earned from donation to pay for school, up from 28 percent from 2002-2004.

In the New York Metropolitan area, most programs see only about 20% of patients who do not have insurance to pay for their IVF cycles. Furthermore, it is estimated that for every patient who does an IVF cycle at least another 2 to 3 would also benefit from the fertility therapy. Unfortunately, for those with an insurance cap and for those paying out of pocket there is an enormous financial pressure for these patients to conceive in the fewest number of cycles to minimize the cost and hence transfer multiple embryos with a resulting increase in multiple pregnancies and the complications of premature deliveries; medical, emotional and financial.

New York State offers a grant for patients in need of IVF that is income based and diminishes the entire cost of the cycle for some lower middle income patients to just a few thousand dollars. However, even this rich program does not cover the cost of frozen embryo transfers and therefore still encourages patients to transfer multiple embryos. Other IVF programs, including my own offer our own income based grant programs and IVF studies significantly reducing the cost of a cycle and making it affordable to nearly everyone in need.

The problem remains that none of these programs discourage patients from "putting all their eggs in one basket" and risking the dangerous multiple pregnancies. Two years ago, I proposed an alternative financial program that does eliminate the financial need to maximize one's chance of conceiving in a single cycle. It is called the Single Embryo Transfer Program at East Coast Fertility. A couple pays the standard $12,000 fee and the egg freezing, storage and frozen embryo transfers are included for an unlimited number of times until they have their baby. I wonder if patients knew about this program if cost would still stand in their way. The beautiful part is we would avoid these risky multiple pregnancies and according to the CDC, in addition to avoiding the medical, emotional and financial hardships caused by the multiple pregnancies, it would save $1billion per year if this program was utilized by all patients who are candidates for it throughout the country.

Yet another side effect of this economic downturn and lack of insurance coverage for IVF has been the fact that patients can have a gonadotropin/IUI cycle for free with a 30 percent risk of multiples and 5 percent risk of triplets or more if their insurance covers it but not the safer IVF alternative where one can control how many embryos to transfer. For patients paying out of pocket many still choose to risk multiples with the less expensive gonadotropin/IUI cycle despite its much lower success rate.

But, all couples don't need a full stimulation IVF cycle. Many couples could try a lower stimulation IVF known as "MicroIVF". The cost of MicroIVF varies but at my program it is offered for example at $3900, approximately the cost of a gonadotropin/IUI cycle and a far cry from the average cost of IVF. MicroIVF does not have the affect on the body that a gonadotropin cycle has nor the high risk of multiple pregnancy. It can be combined with the Single Embryo Transfer Program as well.

It is apparent that we have not done a good enough job communicating to patients about how they can afford fertility treatment with insurance or without. Money can be a barrier to having so many things, let's not make it a barrier for couples to have families. We have to do a better job of letting them know about the solutions that are available to them so that they can afford to get the care that they need to make their dreams of a family come true.

ABC'S OF IVF

It's not all inclusive but perhaps can assist you as a glossary to look up terms as you come across them in your reading

Assisted Hatching is when the embryologist makes a hole in the shell around the embryo called the zona pellucidum. This is performed minutes prior to embryo transfer and may be performed chemically with acid tyrodes, mechanically with a micropipette or with a laser. It is commonly believed that older eggs may lead to embryos with a thicker or harder shell that may prevent the natural hatching of an embryo that must occur prior to the embryo implanting into a woman's lining of her womb.

Blastocyst embryo transfers occur on day 5 or 6 after the egg retrieval. This is the embryonic stage when an embryo normally implants into the womb. These embryos have been selected to be healthier by virtue of the fact that they have made it to this stage.

Some believe that a woman's uterus may be more receptive to an embryo implanted at this stage. Statistically, the pregnancy rates for women who have had blastocysts transferred is higher than when the same number is transferred on day 3 using "cleaved" embryos of 4-10 cells. As the advantage of the blastocyst transfer may be only a matter of selection, it is thought that there may be no advantage if the embryologist is able to select just as well the best embryos to transfer on day 3.

Bravelle – Brand of FSH, follicle stimulating hormone which is a gonadotropin used to stimulate a woman's ovaries to superovulate and make multiple eggs mature during the IVF cycle.

Cetrotide – Brand of Gonadotropin Releasing Hormone Antagonist that prevents a woman's pituitary gland from producing LH, luteinizing hormone. LH increases can trigger premature ovulation and stimulate testosterone and progesterone production which can be harmful to a woman's egg production and prematurely mature the lining of womb potentially affecting implantation.

Co-culture of a woman's endometrial cells from the uterine lining or granulosa cells from aspirated ovarian follicles along with the embryos in the same culture dish is thought to provide growth factors for the embryos which may improve the health and growth of the embryos.

Cleavage Stage Embryos are 2-10 cell embryos transferred on day 2 or 3. They are often graded by their lack of fragmentation and granularity of the inside of the cell cytoplasm; A to D or 1 to 5 with A or 1 being the best grade.

Embryo Glue is a protein supplement to the transfer media prepared minutes prior to transfer to make the embryo more likely to stick to the lining of the womb. It is believed that some embryos may not implant since they are not adhering to the lining and do not get an opportunity to burrow into the endometrium.

Estradiol is produced by the granulosa cells of the follicle which surround the egg in the ovary. As follicles are stimulated and grow they produce more estradiol. We measure estradiol to monitor development of the follicles. It also helps to prepare the lining of the womb for implantation.

Follistim - Brand of FSH, follicle stimulating hormone which is a gonadotropin used to stimulate a woman's ovaries to superovulate and make multiple eggs mature during the IVF cycle.

Ganirelix - Brand of Gonadotropin Releasing Hormone Antagonist that prevents a woman's pituitary gland from producing LH, luteinizing hormone. LH increases can trigger premature ovulation and stimulate testosterone and progesterone production which can be harmful to a woman's egg production and prematurely mature the lining of womb potentially affecting implantation

Gonal F - Brand of FSH, follicle stimulating hormone which is a gonadotropin used to stimulate a woman's ovaries to superovulate and make multiple eggs mature during the IVF cycle.

Gonadotropins - FSH, follicle stimulating hormone and LH, luteinizing hormone stimulate the follicles in the ovary to mature and produce ovarian hormones, estradiol, testosterone and progesterone. It also is used to stimulate a woman's ovaries to superovulate and make multiple eggs mature during the IVF cycle. We adjust the ratio of FSH and LH to achieve goals of optimal follicular development and maturation while trying to minimize the risk of hyperstimulation. Typically we administer the gonadotropins to the woman for 8-14 days before giving her HCG 35-36 hours prior to the egg retrieval

HCG is human chorionic gonadotropin, the pregnancy hormone we measure to see if your wife is pregnant. We follow the numbers to monitor the growth and health of the pregnancy. HCG has the same biological effect as LH and therefore can be used to mature the egg in the same way as if it were getting ready to ovulate. We therefore administer HCG to women 35-36 hours prior to the egg retrieval. Brand names for HCG include Pregnyl and Ovidrel.

HMG – Human Menopausal Gonadotropins are purified from the urine of menopausal women since they have high levels of FSH and LH. Menopur and Repronex are brands of HMG used in IVF stimulations containing a 1:1 ratio of FSH to LH. We adjust the ratio of FSH and LH to achieve goals of optimal follicular development and maturation while trying to minimize the risk of hyperstimulation. Adding pure FSH, i.e. Bravelle, Follistim or Gonal F will increase the ratio of FSH to LH which may be desirable especially early in a stimulation. Some patients may not need any supplemental LH and are stimulated with FSH only. LH is sometimes added towards the end of a stimulation to minimize the risk of hyperstimulation syndrome.

Hyperstimulation syndrome is a condition which occurs approximately 3% of the time as a result of superovulation of a woman's ovaries with gonadotropins. A woman's ovaries become enlarged and cystic; fluid accumulates in her belly, and occasionally around her lungs. When it becomes excessive, it may make it uncomfortable to breathe. We remove this excess fluid with a needle. Women can also become dehydrated and put them at risk of developing blood clots. We therefore recommend fluids high in salt content like V 8 and Campbell's chicken soup. We give patients baby aspirin to prevent clot formation. It may also be recommended to freeze all the embryos and postpone the transfer to a later cycle as pregnancy can significantly exacerbate Hyperstimulation syndrome.

ICSI - Sometimes even in the presence of a normal semen analysis, and normal results on all the infertility tests, fertilization may not occur without microsurgically injecting the sperm directly into the egg. This procedure is called Intracytoplasmic Sperm Injection or ICSI and may achieve fertilization in almost all circumstances where there is otherwise a sperm cause for lack of fertilization

Lupron is a Gonadotropin Releasing Hormone Agonist that must be administered after a woman ovulates or concurrent with progesterone or oral contraceptive pills to effectively suppress gonadotropins. Lupron prevents a woman's pituitary gland from producing LH, luteinizing hormone. LH increases can trigger premature ovulation and stimulate testosterone and progesterone production which can be harmful to a woman's egg production and prematurely mature the lining of womb potentially affecting implantation

Monitoring of a woman's stimulation with gonadotropins is performed by transvaginal ultrasound examination of her ovarian follicles and blood hormone levels. The gonadotropin doses can be adjusted according to the results of the monitoring. The timing of the HCG and subsequent egg retrieval are likewise based on the monitoring. Typically, a woman need not be monitored more frequent than every 3 days initially but may need daily monitoring as she approaches follicular maturation to determine timing of the HCG injection and retrieval.

Morula is the stage between the cleavage stage embryo and blastocyst. It is when the embryo is a ball of cells.

Oral contraceptive pills are often given prior to the stimulation to help time stimulation starts and bring a woman's reproductive system to a baseline state from which the stimulation may be initiated.

Progesterone is an ovarian hormone that prepares the lining of the womb for implantation. We measure it during stimulation to check if the lining is getting prematurely stimulated. We add it to the woman after the retrieval to better prepare the lining and continue it as needed to help sustain the implanted embryo until the placenta takes over production of its own progesterone.

DVD CONTENTS

1. Introduction to Dr. Kreiner
2. Advances in The Field
3. Single Embryo Transfer
4. MicroIVF – Part 1
5. MicroIVF – Part 2
6. High FSH and the Biological Clock
7. Financing Treatment
8. Polycystic Ovarian Syndrome
9. Fibroids
10. Egg Donation
11. Accessibility to Your Doctor
12. Polyps